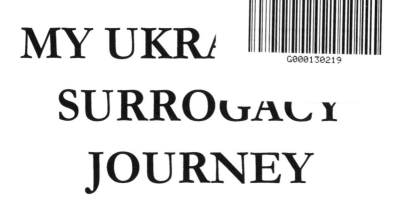

MY UKRAINIAN SURROGACY JOURNEY

A Personal Account of My Mission to Motherhood in Kiev

Bianca Smith

For more information on the author visit

www.wheresmystork.com

Bianca Smith

Also by the same author

IVF A Detailed Guide: Everything I wish I Had Known Before Starting My Fertility Treatments

available on Amazon in eBook & Paperback (in some countries)

& AUDIO (AUDIBLE, AMAZON & iTunes)

The Highs & Lows of my Infertility

Available on Amazon in eBook & Paperback (in some countries)

Cover: **www.loomadesigns.co.za**

Cover photo: **www.facebook.com/sovetoff.photo**

INTRODUCTION: WHY SURROGACY?

Those of you who have been following my story - maybe on my (previous) blog, which has now become a book, *The Highs & Lows of my Infertility* or on my Facebook pages **Where's My Stork? IFV News & Notes**, or **Where's My Stork? Surrogacy News & Notes https://www.facebook.com/surrogacyinfo** or otherwise have read the intro to my previous book *(IVF A Detailed Guide)*, will know that I had been trying to become a mom since 2004, went through miscarriages and 8 rounds of IVF (between July 2013 and April 2016) using own and donor eggs, without any baby to take home.

After my 8th failed round of IVF in April 2016, my husband and I decided to put the baby-making to rest and accept life as a childless couple. However, I just couldn't let it go. The heart wants what the heart wants and no amount of telling myself that we have a great life (which we did and of course still do), would erase that basic longing to be a mother.

We still had one frozen embryo (made with a donor egg) at our last clinic in Prague and we wondered whether we should attempt to make a few more eggs and include a fully donated embryo (donor egg and donor sperm) so that I could give the now "final" transfer a big send off and transfer 3 embryos to my womb instead of just two as I had been doing.

But after all the failures and disappointments, we didn't feel too positive. How would it be different this time? How would transferring one extra embryo suddenly make us pregnant? Over the years we had transferred a total of 13 embryos with no success. We wanted to keep trying to become parents, but it felt like if we just continued to do more of the same, we would continue to get the same disappointing results. So, we concluded that one of the only things we hadn't tried was surrogacy. As it had been several IVF rounds since I had used my own eggs, which we had been told were not so great at that stage already, we settled on exploring donor egg surrogacy.

A few years back, somewhere around IVF cycle number 5, a friend of mine in the UK had offered to be a surrogate for us. As wonderful a gesture as this was, the timing was not right for us and we were still very much on the path of trying to fall pregnant ourselves. Finally, after our 8th unsuccessful IVF, I was warming to the idea of surrogacy. By this time, we had moved to Florida on 5-year visas. Negotiating with a surrogate in the UK while living in Florida did not seem like a viable option. Added to this, was the fact that under UK surrogacy law, anyone who carries and gives birth to a child, regardless of whether her genetics were involved or not, is considered the mother and this woman could decide any time during the pregnancy and after birth to keep the baby. For any couple, but especially for couples who have battled nail, tooth and soul to have their family, this was a frightening thought!

So, I began to research surrogacy in the USA. This research practically came to an end before it had really started. The reason? PRICE! Shock, doesn't even begin to describe the way I felt when looking at all the base numbers presented to me! They were talking over $100k to begin with! Even if we had this kind of money, my husband would have refused to spend that much on something that might yield no return after already spending everything we had and more on all my own treatments! We had just sold our house in the UK and planned to invest the money to make some interest for another house or a business down the line, but I couldn't let go of the idea of the possibility of being a mom through surrogacy. The profit of the sale was £50k and this was our last bit of hope and money to spare on anything. It was - find a surrogacy package for this amount (or less) - or forget the surrogacy idea and our dream of having a family of our own. To make this task even more challenging for me, my husband insisted that I not only find a surrogacy package that fits in with this budget but to find a money-back guarantee in case it fails. He was adamant that without this guarantee, he would not invest in surrogacy. My mission to motherhood continued with renewed determination and hope!

The main reason women turn to surrogacy is due to fertility problems of some kind – whether it is implantation failure of embryos as in my case, repeated miscarriages, or damaged or no womb or a mix of other health problems that can be dangerous for a woman to carry a child. Of course, surrogacy is also used by same sex couples but unfortunately this book is not for those couples as it focuses on Surrogacy in Ukraine and sadly the Ukrainian surrogacy law currently only permits heterosexual (legally married) couples.

Surrogacy these days is done with or without donor eggs and is either traditional or gestational. Traditional Surrogacy means that the woman who will carry the baby gives her own eggs to be joined with the male partner's sperm (or donor sperm). This type of surrogacy is being replaced by *Gestational Surrogacy*, which means that eggs will come from either the intended mother or by an egg donor and then implanted into the womb of another woman who will carry the baby for the couple. In this way, couples who can produce their own embryos but not carry a child can still have their own genetic off-spring. If a couple is using donor eggs, then in gestational surrogacy a separate egg donor and surrogate are used. The idea behind this is that because the surrogate has no genetic link to the baby she is carrying, she will be less likely to want to keep the baby and in some countries such as Ukraine, this is a definite requirement by local surrogacy law.

Overall, surrogacy has had a bad rep all over the world for many reasons. Every time intended parents full of desperate hope flock to another surrogacy-friendly country, anti-surrogacy groups manage to get it shut down – Mexico; India, Cambodia, Thailand and more. There are still modern countries such as the UK and Australia who only allow altruistic surrogacy but are still not that supportive of it - either on home turf or for couples to travel elsewhere to enter surrogacy and so make it an extra difficult and lengthy process for these couples to bring their babies back to their home countries.

WHAT IS THIS BOOK ABOUT & IS IT FOR YOU?

This book is a *personal* account of my experiences, general info, my thoughts and feelings during my surrogacy journey as an intended parent doing surrogacy through a fertility clinic in Kiev, Ukraine. This book discusses our journey from the moment we decided to pursue surrogacy to returning to Florida with our babies; the speed and ease of our journey from deciding on our clinic to navigating the legalities of exiting Ukraine

(British passports for our babies as we are British citizens but live in Florida); our experiences living in Kiev for 4 months, from our clinic's client service to accommodation, shopping and getting around Ukraine; relationship with our surrogate; the birth of our babies; after birth care; travelling back to Florida and various bits and pieces in between, as well as handy resources.

This book is for any **married heterosexual couple:**

*Thinking about pursuing surrogacy in Ukraine. If you have not yet chosen a clinic, then this book is a valuable source of information to add to your research which could help you to make an educated decision.

*If you have already chosen a clinic, then this book could still help your awareness of surrogacy in Kiev in general, as well as prepare you for the pitfalls that you may come across on your journey and assist you in being better equipped to deal with the challenges presented by your clinic, being in a country where close to no English is spoken, where the state medical care is well below the standard that we are used to in other parts of the world and where Brits and Australians (especially but not limited to) need to stay for 2-4 months to await their babies' passports to exit Ukraine while dealing with the already challenging task of being parents (mostly first time parents) to a newborn or two.

Most of the information in this book is based on us being a British couple and therefore following the British surrogacy laws for our exit procedure from Ukraine – obtaining British passports for our babies – and the British Parental Order. However, even if you are from another country, you will still find benefit in a lot of what I have put together – preparations, resources, clinics, doctors, tips from those who have been, what to take with, and so on.

The information in this book is based on my personal journey and I talk honestly and with full transparency about all my experiences – both good and bad. I am not telling you to go or not to go to Ukraine for your surrogacy journey – that is up to you to decide after weighing up all the pros and cons relating to your own journey and what will be best for you as intended parents and what you are prepared to put up with vs what best suits your budget.

This book is not meant to slander any country, city, organization or person and therefore should not be read as such. It is a personal record so please take it as it is intended. Also, no two journeys are the same. My experiences don't necessarily dictate how other people's experiences will be.

The clinics and service providers mentioned in this book are based on my own preference and experiences or those of other ladies/couples on this journey that I have spoken to, and not on any documented statistics.

Please note that I have not received any sort of compensation from any service provider mentioned in this book as part of paid advertising or any other promotion whatsoever.

I hope that you will find this book useful and I wish you all the luck in the world on your journey. It's not an easy journey but equipping yourself with as much knowledge as possible is always guaranteed to help make life at least a little easier, and that's what I am trying to do for you through this book.

I would like to thank everyone who was involved in any way in my life in a positive manner – my husband, my friends, the many ladies in all my on-line support groups and my family, as well as everyone who was involved in the creation of this book.

With love,

Bianca

TABLE OF CONTENTS   PG

CHAPTER 1 – CHOOSING UKRAINE FOR SURROGACY

In July 2016, I got to work searching for a surrogacy clinic that we could afford (with our 50K that we had made from our UK house sale) *and* that had a money back guarantee. I had never favoured surrogacy before and therefore had absolutely no idea where to start. Although I had been in fertility groups for 4 years and had done extensive research on everything IVF, I found the information on surrogacy to be very vague. I did not know any intended parents or surrogates and all info I was getting was from someone that knew someone somewhere down the line. I began to make phone calls across the USA, almost like travelling the ocean from Africa to Australia in a rubber dinghy. Most surrogacy agencies I spoke to were instantly dismissive when I enquired about a money-back guarantee. Some of them rudely laughed in my face and told me that I was crazy and shouldn't even be thinking about surrogacy if I didn't at least have $80,000 to start with. With every phone call, my hopes and dreams of motherhood shattered even further. My next lot of research focused on Mexico, which seemed ideal – affordable, beautiful and only a quick hop over from our home in Florida – perfect! Except, I discovered, Mexico had just shut down legal surrogacy and it was now a no-go zone. Sadly, we had just missed our window of opportunity for surrogacy in Mexico. However, somewhere in this chaos there was a glimmer of hope. After one agency informed me about their clinic in Mexico shutting down, they suggested that I try some of the only countries still allowing legal surrogacy – Russia and Ukraine. Here I thought I was rather knowledgeable about fertility tourism in Europe, but I had no idea that either Russia or Ukraine offered tourist fertility treatments (including surrogacy) of any kind. So, my fingers hit the keyboard for continued research and hope!

Before long I was overjoyed to find a Russian agency that fitted exactly into our budget AND offered a percentage of our money back after three failed attempts! This was hitting the triple 7 jackpot in the surrogacy gamble! That was until… I found a surrogacy support group on Facebook and someone mentioned that Ukraine offered something even better – an unlimited package guarantee! A What?! Unlimited package until you go home with a baby?! I contacted the agency immediately. Two days later I received all their information and spent the next 200 hours lapping up this info hoping it didn't burst into flame before my eyes!

We set a visit to the clinic in Kiev for our earliest possible availability, which was 3 months later in October 2016. Read more about this in my collection of blog posts, *The Highs & Lows of my Infertility*.

CHAPTER 2 – PREPARING FOR OUR INITIAL SURROGACY CONSULTATION

We had three months before our initial consultation with the clinic in Kiev, which meant that we had three months to prepare my husband's swimmers for tip top performance to qualify for the unlimited guarantee package.

Here is the full list of requirements and test results needed by our clinic to qualify for the (unlimited) surrogacy package:

1 As already mentioned, surrogacy in Ukraine is only for **legally married heterosexual** couples (all Ukraine).

2 Intended Parents (IP's) must provide **medical reports or a letter from a**

medical professional confirming that they are not able to carry a child of their own due to medical reasons such as:

-Absence of a womb

-Deformation of the uterus, making pregnancy and delivery impossible

-Adhesions of womb cavity which cannot be healed

-Somatic diseases which prevent carrying a pregnancy to avoid putting a woman's health or life at risk

-Unsuccessful IVF attempts (at least 4) with good quality embryos

3 **Marriage certificate which must be certified or apostilled** (see this webpage for a further explanation on apostille **www.internationalapostille.com/what-is-an-apostille**)

4 **Passports** (with a **coloured** photo copy of **every** page for the **British** passport application)

Husband

5 Sperm count

6 Chest X-Ray (these can be done cheap and easy in Kiev)

7 Blood group and Rh-factor

8 Blood test results for HIV, hepatitis B & C, Syphilis

9 Karyotype test results

Wife if using OWN eggs

10 Doctor's letter stating that it is safe for you to proceed with hormonal

ovarian stimulation

11 Any medical records pertaining to previous fertility treatments –
IUI/IVF/egg donation attempts and why surrogacy is recommended

12 Breast ultrasound results if under 50 and no previous breast problems –
otherwise mammogram results

13 Latest transvaginal ultrasound results

14 Blood test results for your LH, FSH, Progesterone, Oestrogen,
Testosterone and AMH levels

15 Chest X-Ray (these can be done cheap and easy in Kiev)

16 Blood group and Rh-factor

17 Blood test results for HIV, hepatitis B & C, Syphilis

18 Karyotype test results

19 Any other medical records in support of your medical case

If using DONOR EGGS, you will only need your medical letter stating
your reasons for pursuing surrogacy and any previous IUI/IVF records as
mentioned in the beginning of the document list.

*** *NOTE: All these documents should be scanned and
emailed to your agency before your first visit & the
originals taken with you to your first visit* ***

As we had decided to go straight for donor egg surrogacy (due to my own eggs having a bad rep already back in 2014), the full focus the next three months was on my husband, Vinny. We got to work doing everything that we could in our own power to improve the quality, quantity and mobility of his sperm.

Note:

Sperm are living cells and therefore get affected by everything that the body is exposed to – chemicals in the air or food, extreme temperatures, drugs (prescription and recreational), smoking, and diet, which will either improve their health or cause degeneration.

The good news is that many times even if they have been exposed to negative factors, the result can be reversed. This will take between 2.5 and 3 months of healthy living for the sperm to regenerate as well as mature enough to fertilise an egg.

The following is how my husband prepared for the next 3 months to improve his sperm count, quality and mobility:

STRICTLY NO to

#Non-stick cookware

#Soy

#Wheat

#Sugar

#Dairy

#Pork

#Meat with hormones

#Alcohol

#Trans fats

#Processed foods of any kind

#Food from tin cans

#Fish with exceptions (see below)

#Mobile phone in pocket or near testes

#Computer on lap or near testes

#Heat near testes

#Plastic food storage containers

#Tight-fitting underwear

#Exposure to chemicals from toiletries, household cleaners and sunscreen

#Cash receipts (which are laced in harmful fertility destroying chemicals)

#Food or drinks out of plastic

YES to

ONLY olive or coconut oil

ONLY Snapper, Salmon and Cod fish not more than once a week

ONLY organic products

ONLY filtered water (no water from plastic bottles)

Cast iron cookware preferable

Marble cutting board preferable to wood (NOT plastic)

Wash all vegetables well

Try to eliminate as many toxic products in the house as possible - ONLY

ALL-NATURAL cleaning products & personal hygiene products

Supplements (see list below)

Eat MOSTLY…

Vitamin C

- Red peppers
- Broccoli
- Cranberries
- Potatoes
- Tomatoes
- Citrus Fruit

Vitamin E

- Sunflower seeds
- Peanuts (and peanut butter)
- Almonds
- Spinach/ kale
- Papaya
- Dark leafy greens

Folate

- Liver
- Beans (no tin cans)

Vitamin B12

- Lamb
- Beef
- Eggs

Zinc

- Calf liver

- Raw pumpkin seeds
- Turkey
- Peanuts (and peanut butter)

Selenium

- Brazil nuts
- Snapper / salmon / cod / shrimp

OTHER FOODS Known for Detoxing and Anti-Inflammatory properties)

- Fresh ginger
- Banana
- Almond milk
- Peanut butter
- Onions
- Avocado
- Basil
- Coconut Oil (see this blog for more info on the benefits of coconut oil **https://wellnessmama.com/5734/coconut-oil**)
- Flaxseed (see this link for the amazing benefits of Flaxseed **www.organicfacts.net/health-benefits/seed-and-nut/health-benefits-of-flaxseed.html**)

SUPPLEMENTS

Most important

- Zinc

- CoQ10
- Vitamin E
- Vitamin B12
- L'Caritine
- Vitamin C&D
- Folate
- Tribulus
- Selenium
- Lipoic Acid
- Melatonin
- Royal Jelly

Other

- American Ginseng Root
- Ashwagandha Root
- Fo-ti
- Ginko leaves
- Goji Berries
- Maca Root
- Schisandra

This is a very strict regime and although my hubby was surprisingly dedicated (he used to love his processed food!), there were tough moments but if your hubby perseveres (with your loving encouragement), the results will speak for themselves. Most of you who have reached this point have been through the craziness of fertility treatments repeatedly, year after year, so if 3 hard months of dedication to your diet and lifestyle can bring you the baby you have dreamt of for years, then wouldn't it be worth every bit of sugary snack or cheese toasty that your hubby is not putting in his body?! Small price to pay after the thousands of $ down the drain, countless needles in the belly, crazy-witch inducing hormones…ok, you get my point! This worked for us and we swear by it!

Also, you can have fun with this and see how many tasty, new recipes you can come up with! Ladies, if you help your hubby by putting your best chef hat on, then he might not even feel like he's missing out on anything! *Here's a few of my own recipe creations to get you started.*

NOTE:

All these recipes can of course be adjusted to your personal tastes – if you love onions, add another or if you're not that keen on garlic, use 3 cloves instead of 6 (or even none) and so on. My husband and I love spicy food so I'm heavy on the spices and as you will see, most of these dishes include my go-to main spices of paprika, curry powder and turmeric (see the benefits of turmeric here **www.healthline.com/nutrition/top-10-evidence-based-health-benefits-of-turmeric**).

So, use my recipes as a base and play around to see what works for you by mixing and matching quantities and ingredients from the list above. Note that all the ingredients should be ORGANIC and preferably cooked in cast iron pots and pans.

GARLICKY POTATO COD (rich in Selenium, Vitamin C & Vitamin E)

Bianca Smith

Ingredients

2 Fresh or frozen cod loins

1 Medium onion – chopped

6 Cloves fresh garlic – chopped

1 Small red pepper – chopped

2 Tomatoes

3 Medium potatoes – boiled

2 Large handfuls fresh spinach/chard or dark leafy greens

2 Tablespoons ground flaxseed

3 Tablespoons curry powder

2 Tablespoons paprika

2 Tablespoons turmeric

1 Tablespoon ginger

Sprinkling Italian herbs

Sprinkling salt and pepper

Method

1 Heat coconut oil in cast iron wok or pot

2 Add onions and garlic until browned

3 Add red pepper

4 Fry for a few minutes on high heat, stirring continuously

5 Cut the raw cod fillets in strips and add to the wok

6 Cook for a further few minutes then reduce to a medium heat

7 Cut the boiled potatoes in medium chunks and add to the wok

8 Add the flaxseed, herbs, spices, salt and pepper

9 Squeeze the juice from the tomatoes into the mixture then cut the pulp into pieces and add to mix

10 Reduce to a lower heat, stir fry for 5 minutes then add the fresh dark leaves and stir fry for a further 10 minutes – keep stirring

BASIL TURKEY BURGER PATTIES (rich in zinc)

Ingredients

Ground turkey (I use around 500 grams/ 1 lb for two of us)

2 Tablespoons ground flaxseed

2 Tablespoons ginger

2 Tablespoons turmeric

2 Tablespoons paprika

Sprinkling Italian herbs

Sprinkling salt & pepper

2 Large handfuls fresh basil

Method

1 Mix everything together with hands in a stainless-steel or ceramic bowl

2 Divide into 4 balls

3 Grease-proof a cast iron or ceramic baking dish with either olive or coconut oil

4 Put balls into dish, flatten slightly and add ground salt to the top of each

5 Bake at 350 degrees F/ 180 degrees C for 15 min on each side

PAPRIKA INFUSED KALE LAMB BURGERS

(rich in Vitamin B12, Vitamin E and folate)

Ingredients

Ground lamb (for two)

1 Medium onion - chopped

6 Cloves fresh garlic – chopped

2 Large handfuls kale

2 Tablespoons paprika

2 Tablespoons curry powder

2 Tablespoons turmeric

2 Tablespoons ground flaxseed

Half cup lemon juice

Sprinkling salt & pepper

Method

1 Brown the onion and garlic in coconut oil and then add the kale to soften

2 Allow to cool

3 Mix everything together with hands in a stainless-steel or ceramic bowl

4 Divide into 4 balls

5 Grease-proof a cast iron or ceramic baking dish with either olive or coconut oil

6 Put balls into dish, flatten slightly and add ground salt to the top of each

7 Bake at 350 degrees F for 15 min on each side

Curried Peanut Butter Chicken (rich in Vitamin C, Vitamin E, Selenium and Zinc)

Ingredients

2 Chicken breasts – cut into chunks

2 Tablespoons peanut butter

1 Medium onion - chopped

6 Cloves garlic – whole or chopped

2 Tablespoons ground flaxseed

2 Tablespoons turmeric

2 Tablespoons curry powder

2 Tablespoons paprika

2 Tablespoons ground ginger

1 Large handful dried cranberries

1 Large handful walnuts - chopped

1 Large handful sunflower seeds

2 Potatoes – cut into chunks

1 Cup almond milk

Method

1 Brown the onion and garlic in the coconut oil in a cast iron pot

2 Add the turmeric, curry powder, paprika and ginger – keep stirring to ensure that nothing burns and that all the onion and garlic is coated

3 Add the chicken chunks and keep stirring and coating the chunks in the spices

4 Add the peanut butter and keep stirring

5 Transfer to a casserole pot (preferably cast iron)

6 Add the cranberries, walnuts, sunflower seeds, and potato

7 Bake in the oven at 350 degrees F for 40 minutes or until the potatoes are soft

Nutty Beef

(rich in Vitamin B12, Vitamin E, Vitamin C, Zinc and Selenium)

Ingredients

Ground beef (for two)

1 Medium onion - chopped

6 Cloves garlic - chopped

2 Tablespoons curry powder

2 Tablespoons turmeric

2 Tablespoons Paprika

2 Tablespoons ground flaxseed

Half a cup of lemon juice

1 Tablespoon peanut butter

2-4 Large fresh tomatoes

1 Handful of sunflower seeds

1 Handful mixed nuts

1 Handful dried cranberries

1 Handful of kale

Method

1 Brown the chopped onion and garlic in coconut oil in a cast iron pot

2 Add the ground beef and brown

3 Add all the spices and keep stirring to make sure all is well coated

4 Stir in the flaxseed

5 Add lemon juice, squeeze the juice from the tomatoes and then break pulp into mix

6 Add the sunflower seeds, nuts and cranberries

7Simmer for 10 min

8 Add peanut butter and simmer for a further 5 min

9 Add kale and simmer for a last 5 min

Cashew Ground Turkey (rich in Vitamin D, Vitamin E, Zinc and Folate)

Ingredients

Ground turkey (for two)

1 Medium Onion - chopped

6 Cloves garlic - chopped

1-2 Cups mushrooms - chopped

2 Tablespoons turmeric

2 Tablespoons ground ginger

1 Handful sunflower seeds

1 Cup cashew milk

Ground flaxseed

2 Large handfuls spinach, pak choy and mustard green mix (or similar)

1-2 Red peppers

1 Cup quinoa

Sprinkling of chopped cashews

Course sea or Himalayan salt

Method

1 Sauté onions and garlic in coconut oil in cast iron wok or pot

2 Add mushrooms and stir fry, cooking on high heat to get rid of moisture

3 Add the spices

4 Add the turkey and brown

5 Mix well and cook on high for 4 min - keep stirring

6 Add the sunflower seeds and cashew milk

7 Reduce heat and simmer for 10 min

8 Add the flaxseed – simmer for another 5 min

9 Add the greens – simmer for a further 5 min

11 <u>To cook the Quinoa – I use a ready pack for speed and convenience – follow the directions on your pack. What I usually do is</u>:

Measure out 1 cup quinoa into a sieve and rinse thoroughly

Heat a few spoons of coconut oil in a cast iron pot and then add the rinsed quinoa

Fry for a few minutes continuously stirring to make sure that it doesn't burn

Then add 3 cups of (filtered) water to the pot

Once it is boiling, reduce heat and simmer for 30 minutes or until there is no more moisture in the pot – be careful that you don't run out of water or it will burn

Then combine the Quinoa and Turkey mixture

12 Coat the whole red pepper in coconut oil place onto a baking tray and grill for roughly 20 minutes on each side or until "blackened" then cut the peppers into halves

13 Spoon the mixture into each pepper half

14 Sprinkle with the salt, cashew crumbles and drizzle with coconut oil

For delicious variations on shakes, try:

Breakfast Orange Shake

Ingredients:

Orange juice

Kale

Banana

Mix all in a blender to start your day with some natural Vitamin E, Vitamin C and Folate

Get-up-and-go Almond Shake

<u>Ingredients</u>:

Almond milk

Banana

Peanut butter

Mix all in a blender for a breakfast loaded with energy, Vitamin E and Zinc

Sugar-Free, Dairy-Free Decadent Chocolate Pudding (rich in Vitamin E and Zinc)

<u>Ingredients</u>:

3Bananas

Quarter cup raw unsweetened Cocoa

Half cup natural sugar-free Peanut or Almond butter

Handful of chopped nuts of your choice for some crunch (I use walnuts)

2 Tablespoons organic and sugar-free vanilla essence

<u>Method</u>:

1 Add all the ingredients to a stainless-steel bowl and mix with an electronic mixer on high speed

2 Spoon in a glass dish and refrigerate

Variation to the above: Spoon into a baking dish that has been greased with coconut oil and bake for 20 minutes on 350 degrees F / 180 degrees C. Once it has cooled, cut into squares and freeze them for on-the-go-snacks when you feel like a little healthy sweetness

CHAPTER 3 - INITIAL CONSULTATION WITH OUR CLINIC IN KIEV

On the 15th of October 2016 (incidentally, that happens to be worldwide baby loss remembrance day), we boarded a plane from Tampa, Florida to Kiev, Ukraine full of excitement and rattled nerves.

We had a sleepless 8-hour flight from Tampa to London, a few hours wait at Gatwick for our sleepless 3.5-hour flight to Kiev and an exhausting (and harrowing) hour long drive to our hotel.

There is no direct flight from Tampa to Kiev, so we travelled direct to Gatwick on British Airways and to Kiev on Air Ukraine. EU nationals and Americans (and some other countries) do not need a visa to enter Ukraine for 90 days. You only need a valid passport, which will be stamped as you enter.

A driver from our clinic met us at the airport and took us to the clinic-owned hotel, where we were taken to a reasonably sized room to drop off our things before dinner. Dinner was in a separate part of the hotel in a dining hall and was a buffet of mixed western and Ukrainian dishes, including unlimited ice-creams (sometimes it's the small things, right?).

Jetlag hit us with racing minds from 3 to 6 in the morning, Has Vinny's strict diet worked? Will we be approved for our unlimited tries/baby guarantee package? Will this trip be the start of our baby dreams finally coming true or had we just added an extra expense to our already blown out of the water budget? There is no budget when it comes to assisted reproduction! Sure, you start off with one but if it doesn't work the first, second, third, fourth time, many of us will choose to only eat dry bread once a week to save for the next shot at being parents. It is indeed a gamble with high stakes – money, mind, emotions and body could all be ruined for no win at all. But I digress…

After a very filling feast of pancakes and pastries (just me, as Vinny had to fast for his blood tests – one advantage of using donor eggs – every cloud with its silver lining and such ha), a driver took us in a minivan to the clinic. Our fluent English-speaking coordinator met us at reception and directed us to a lounge where hordes of other couples filled in forms, sat around chatting, waiting to do their blood or sperm tests, stuffed their faces with tasty treats and drank copious amounts of coffee. One thing they all had in common was the look of hope on their faces!

Vinny went off to do his blood tests (HIV, Hep B, Hep C and Syphilis) as well as give his first sperm deposit. This was the moment that we had been prepping for – had his sperm made the grade?! Finally, our coordinator returned to give us the good news – in her own words "We can totally work with your sperm"! What a relief! Those three months of sacrifice that Vinny had made abstaining from everything he enjoyed eating or drinking really paid off. We were accepted into the unlimited/ guarantee package and we would be getting our much-wanted baby sooner or later! I can't even describe the happiness we felt already!

We then met with the doctor in charge of the egg donors and while we sat there, details of a new egg donor came in who apparently looked just like me! None of the staff could believe the striking resemblance. They showed us a photo and she did look like me as far as we could tell from that one photo.

We spent the next few hours going through and signing our contracts. As this was our final push to bring a baby home, we decided to go all out and make this an awesome experience by choosing the VIP package.

Here is the package we signed for:

ALL INCLUSIVE VIP PACKAGE 49,900 EUROS (ROUGHLY $62,000 OR £44,000)

#Accommodation in a separate apartment provided by the clinic

#All food cooked on premises by a housekeeper to match the standard of food at the hotel accommodation ***

#Services of a personal driver with a vehicle ***

#A smartphone and a Ukrainian SIM card for communication ***

#The services of an interpreter throughout the program

#Needed blood tests are performed by a nurse in the apartment where the Intended Parents are staying

#All medical services needed to achieve pregnancy, including medical examination & tests for Intended Parents throughout the program

#The Intended Parents are provided with PGD service to detect the possible genetic abnormalities. If needed the sex of a baby may be detected (for medical reasons only)

#A Surrogate who has had already had a successful previous surrogacy pregnancy and birth ***

#Miscarriage, abortion or death at any time during the program, reattempts will be covered fully by the clinic on this package

#In case of premature birth all the expenses related to additional medical treatment and special medical equipment utilization shall be covered by the clinic from the first day of birth

#The Intended Parents can stay in the specially equipped maternity house (hospital) together with a baby ***

#The Intended Parents are provided with a new-born package – all the things needed to take care of a newborn baby

#The Intended Parents are provided with a complete physical check-up of the baby by specialists ***

#The Intended Parents are provided with a paediatrician who shall visit the baby every day. A 24/7 phone consultation with a leading English-speaking paediatrician will also be available. If needed the leading paediatrician will visit the baby upon request. ***

#The services of a babysitter from 9am to 6pm

#No additional charge for twins

#Preparation and signing of the contract between surrogate and Intended Parents

#Preparation and signing the contract between the clinic and Intended Parents

#Coordination and monitoring of all personal documents throughout the program

#Coordination and Supervision of the full Surrogacy program until the birth of the baby and the preparation of the necessary documents for the baby to return home with the parents

#The clinic will provide information via email on the surrogate's pregnancy at least once a month

#DNA tests to confirm parenthood in a clinic appointed laboratory

#Submission of the documents concerning the birth certificate of the child to the Ukrainian Civil Registry Office, where the names of the Intended

Parents are indicated. Translation and legalization of the birth certificate are also included

#Assistance to the Intended Parents in obtaining a passport/travel pass in the name of the child

#All medical procedures for the surrogate

#Psychological and physical testing for the surrogate to ensure that she is in a fit state for pregnancy and delivery of a healthy baby

#All ultrasounds and medical care for the surrogate throughout the pregnancy

#Weekly check-up by the clinic (by phone or visit) of the surrogate's health and needs during her pregnancy including any medical examinations

#Medical insurance for the surrogate in case of unforeseen circumstances

#Birth of the baby

#In case of miscarriage, abortion or death *before* 12 weeks, then the clinic will cover the expenses of reattempts - time periods before additional attempts will be determined by the doctor only.

#Transportation, accommodation in a private room and meals for the surrogate ***

#Payment to the Surrogate for pregnancy and birth

EXCLUSIONS:

Transportation from own country to Kiev

All the expenses related to the processing of papers by the relevant Embassies and issuance of the travel documents/passports by these authorities

Payment Schedule for the VIP Package

First instalment: **10,000** EUROS – First visit to the clinic after signing the contracts

Second instalment: **9,900** EUROS - Second visit to the clinic before fertilisation

Third instalment: **10,000** EUROS – After the 12-week ultrasound

Fourth instalment: **10,000** EUROS – After the birth of the child before paper processing

Fifth Instalment: **10,000** EUROS – After receiving baby's birth certificate & on day of embassy appointment. Any additional documents required by the embassy are prepared after the final payment is made. ***

*** It is important to note at this time, that what we signed in our VIP package contract is NOT fully what we received from the agency/clinic. Do read on before you decide on choosing a clinic to find out what service

we received further down the line.

That afternoon we were taken back to the hotel for a buffet dinner and much needed sleep!

The following day we had a fun time going through the egg donor potentials. We were given a 2-week access to the donor egg data base of around 200 women of all shapes, sizes and looks. Most Slavic looks are blond, fair skin with light eyes, so it was easy to find a match for my own fair European looks. Each donor had a profile detailing basic features – hair, eyes, weight, height, age, etc. with photos and 360-degree 3D pics as well as videos of them speaking about themselves with English subtitles.

We made a shortlist of 4 women in order of preference and emailed them to our program coordinator.

Because we had chosen the VIP package, that evening they moved us from the hotel to our own apartment with a live-in housekeeper who cleaned, did our washing and cooked 3 full traditional Ukrainian meals a day. It was strange having a live-in housekeeper, but we thought perhaps we would appreciate it once we had a baby to take care of.

Wednesday morning the driver collected us to take us to the clinic for Vinny to give another sperm deposit. The plan was to give multiple deposits and freeze them in case of failures then we didn't have to fly over to Ukraine again until we came for our baby's birth. The clinic was just as crazy and busy and the wait just as long as it had been on Monday.

Thursday, we attempted to go sightseeing in Kiev, but this was the middle of October and I am a sun worshipper so trying to have fun in 4 degrees

Celsius was no easy task for me. My body started shutting down and I was miserable! So, we decided to do the big red tourist bus but while waiting for the bus, I decided to warm up with a few Irish Coffees meaning that I was bursting for a tinkle in the middle of our bus ride. The tour guide (or just ticket taker, as the guide was one of those things you plug into in and listen to on earpieces that hurt the ears) advised us that there was a toilet in the park at the next stop. To my horror, the steps of the toilets led to an underground hole. Yes! Just a hole to squat over! Nothing else! Even for the woman! And oh, the stench!!

On another attempt to sightsee a few days later we got lost in town and while we were trying to figure out where we were, a friendly 'bear' came to help with directions, which led to a half hour conversation about where we were from, photos with the bear and a fee of a few hundred Ukrainian Hryvnas. We discovered that the place we were looking for (Maidan Square) was the next street up and was filled with not only men in bear suits, but men in cat and Disney suits as well looking to make a few hundred Hryvnas or dollars or pounds – whatever they could get. Scammed! Ha! But it was a good laugh and created fun memories.

Friday, we went back to the clinic for Vinny's last sperm deposit and were told that they had found us a surrogate. Also, if we agreed to use the new egg donor whom everyone had said looked just like me then we were good to go immediately. If we wanted to use one of the other 4 ladies from our shortlist, then we would have to wait. After 13 years of wanting to be a mom and 4 years of failed IVF treatments, and me already 42 years old, there was no way we wanted to wait a minute longer! So, without knowing anything about the egg donor except her general looks and age, we agreed to go for it! Egg collection would be in three weeks on 9 November and transfer 5 days after that on 14 November! There were absolutely no words to describe the excitement, hope, happiness and nervous energy we felt at that moment!

We left Kiev at the end of the week with a light in our eyes that had disappeared a few IVF's back! We knew this was it! The universe's deliveries had been sent out and soon we would receive our precious package we had been waiting so long for!

Discoveries/ Highlights from our First Visit to Kiev

@We met a wonderful Australian couple on a similar journey to us that we are still in contact with.

@Vodka is cheaper than water, costs a few pennies and there are aisles and aisles of bottles to choose from!

@The language is Cyrillic, which makes it very difficult to read. Google translate has a hard time translating accurately between Ukrainian and English so opt for Russian instead.

@October is the start of a very cold winter!

@Driving and rules either don't exist here or are just completely ignored – speed, recklessness, driving through red lights and nearly running pedestrians over on crossings! Learn to be streetwise and follow the lead of the locals when crossing!

@The food is very starchy, there are no preservatives, most things are made from scratch and in general is so different from ours. We had a bowl of cheesy mash for breakfast! Weird!

@There are no tumble dryers so unless your heating is on, then your washing will take days to dry.

@Speaking of heating – the central heating is controlled by the government and is only switched on some time in the middle of October.

@You want to avoid public toilets as best you can, especially in a park. I've also heard that McDonald's is a no go too. It's worth spending on a drink in a bar to use those facilities, which are most often clean.

CHAPTER 4 – THE NEXT FEW MONTHS (of Pregnancy)

We left Kiev full of renewed hope and optimism that our baby dreams were finally about to come true!

How things unfolded

#9 November 2016, our egg donor had her collection

#14 November 2016, our surrogate had her embryo transfer and we received the report later that afternoon telling us that 9 eggs had been collected and 3 grade AA blastocysts had been transferred to our surrogate via ICSI.

#28 November 2016 we received an email from the agency/clinic telling us that our surrogate was pregnant with a beta score of 2367

#14 December 2016 date we received a report from our surrogate's viability scan telling us that we had two strong heartbeats!!!

#31 January 2017, our surrogate had her dating scan at 13 weeks pregnant. We were given 7 August as the due date. It was now that we were also told that we had two boys! - **www.wheresmystork.com/donor-surrogate-dad-wannabee-mom-2-mini-vinnies**

#This was also the first time that we were permitted by the agency/clinic to get any information about our surrogate. We found out her name and age (27). Apparently from this time forward, intended parents can attend all the ultrasounds in person or have a skype call with their surrogate each month when she goes into the clinic for an ultrasound. As we live in America, it was way too far and expensive for us to travel to Kiev for this, but unfortunately the agency/clinic failed to tell us that we could skype instead. (*We only found this out from another intended parent in a passing comment when our surrogate was 30 weeks pregnant!*)

#From here on, we received monthly reports on how the boys were doing at various stages with results of the Nuchal Translucency tests at 13 weeks and the triple screen tests at 18 weeks, as well as ultrasound updates (pictures and videos where we could see their heartbeats (unfortunately the videos had no sound, so we couldn't hear them).

#We managed to have two 5-minute Skype chats with our surrogate through a translator, which was nerve wracking – all of us full of nervous energy and feeling very shy! Vinny and I were also a little sleep deprived. The excitement of the upcoming call kept me up all night and Vinny was half asleep as we had to connect at 3am due to the time difference. Here in Florida, we are 7 hours behind Kiev time.

Our Preparations

@During this time, we tried to do everything possible to not only prepare for parenthood but to enjoy all the stages of our surrogate's pregnancy by ensuring that we celebrated every single milestone. Whenever we received an updated ultrasound or report, we would go out for a meal and talk about that stage of development - **www.wheresmystork.com/our-boys-are-growing-18-weeks-today**

@I wrote a few letters to my boys in my blog according to how I was feeling at that moment and as a form of connecting to our babies in a spiritual sense - **www.wheresmystork.com/letter-1-to-my-surrogate-twin-boys**

@I started collecting gifts for our surrogate and her two little girls. <u>The gift pack included</u>:

*A pretty necklace which was a birds' nest charm of silver-plated wire with 2 blue eggs in and I personalized it by including a "thank you" from Max & Alex (our boys).

*A collection of pampering indulgences from Bath & Body Works – I assumed they would be welcome especially after a twin pregnancy.

*A bottle of designer perfume

*British collections – luxury boxes of tea and edibles for mom and purses and trinkets for her girls

*Shorts & tops with American logos and toys for the little girls

@We downloaded a bunch of parenting books of all styles and recommendations on Audible and listened to them every time we had a spare moment – at the gym, driving to work or lying by the pool.

@We waded into the deep ocean of legal paperwork and processes that we would need to get our babies home to Florida and legally ours – Exiting from Kiev which meant British passports for the boys (as we are British nationals), applying for and obtaining the required Parental Order (also British surrogacy law) and getting American visas for our boys to return to America with us. We spent many days and weeks researching website after website. We also had a Skype consultation with Natalie Gamble Associates which cost us £650 and included a written report about our conversation. Within this consultation, they confirmed that they could not assist us with the passport applications as, number one, they cannot apply on our behalf because application must be made in person by all applicants and number two, they can do nothing to speed up the receipt of the passports. Their expertise lies in the Parental Order process in which they quoted us £20K for the full house package, £5k PLUS expenses for the support package in which they will send our application to the court, prepare all the docs for the surrogate to sign, prepare a first draft of statements for us to expand on, list all the documents needed to submit to the court, draft an index for our court bundle to give us an idea of how to put everything together, and advice how to arrange a meeting with the court representative and court hearings. The third option was an hourly rate for any help we needed of which they advised to budget a minimum of £2k. After spending an absolute fortune on all our fertility treatments over the last 4 years and now for surrogacy, and because we really hadn't thought of budgeting for legal fees, my husband (much to my own discontentment) put his foot down and absolutely refused to pay anyone to do this for us. So, at the time of writing, we managed to arrive safely back in Tampa, Florida with our boys and their British passports without any solicitor's help, and we have received our first court date, been in contact with our Court appointed social worker and submitted our Court statements and evidence, without any outside assistance. **Read on for detailed information on our passport and parental order procedure.**

@We enjoyed date nights, parties with friends and last childless couple experiences, as well as a baby shower aka "go get our boys" BBQ!

CHAPTER 5 – PREPARING TO MEET OUR BABIES IN KIEV, UKRAINE

The day before the 4th of July, I kissed my little feline twins goodbye with a sad heart to be leaving them for so long, but also full of excitement for everything that was to come!

We flew British Airways direct from Tampa to London Gatwick and spent the next 4 days arranging the necessary paperwork (affidavit, apostille, birth certificates – basically everything we needed for passport and parental order applications).

You might want to check out my You Tube update at this point – me talking from our first stop – the UK

https://youtu.be/L2xJpD-ZCE4

Saturday 8 July, we flew from London to Kiev. An agency driver took us to our apartment, after having to call to find out where he was. *It must be noted that we were not taken to the address that we were given a few days before. We had especially asked the agency's project manager to give us the exact address as my in-laws were coming to visit us and wanted to book a hotel within walking distance to our apartment. We explained this to the manager a few days before but were taken to a different apartment many miles away!* This was the start of a series of troubles with the agency while we were in Kiev.

The apartment was big but still only had only 2 bedrooms, ours and the babies' (we have heard from other IP's also on the VIP package that they were given a 4-bedroom apartment to stay in!). The strangest thing was that we had a live-in housekeeper who slept on the couch in the lounge?! A live-in maid? And a live-in maid that lives on the couch?! Very odd! She informed us through google translate that her bed time was at 10pm – talk about a blatant hint!

For the next week we tried to be out of the apartment as much as possible so that we could have space without the housekeeper there, sitting on the couch in the lounge watching Ukrainian TV all day and night. When the agency finally granted our request for privacy, we discovered for the first time that the apartment did have a bunch of English TV channels! This was not the only thing that we discovered…!

When this housekeeper eventually left from the couch, and we had the apartment to ourselves, we were shocked to discover that the whole kitchen/lounge area was a filthy disgrace! All her clothes, underclothes, toiletries, including feminine products were stuffed throughout the lounge. But this wasn't the worst.

We discovered that everything in the kitchen was coated with raw meat fat – like she had made meatballs with her hands then touched every item in the kitchen and never wiped it off. Some of the dishes had never been washed. The trash in the cupboard under the sink had overflowed and never been removed. There were rotten vegetable skins and fruit squashed against the cupboard and covered in mould. All the cutlery in the drawer had been used and just put back dirty with whatever they had cut still stuck to them. The plates, mixing bowls and pots had also been put away without being washed. The bread bin was full of blue mouldy pieces of bread and toast. So, in other words, the housekeeper was serving the same toast every day – what was not eaten kept being put back in the bread bin! The fridge was filthy with open meat just thrown in – no container or covering. Half cans of food were left open in the fridge way past their expiry date. There were several open milk bottles – all growing with age. On the little balcony where washing should be hung, was an overflowing ashtray. Why did we even have a housekeeper who smoked (especially in the apartment) when we were getting newborns?! On closer inspection, the entire apartment was filthy.

We made this grim discovery on a Friday and immediately let the managers and department head know about it. We received no message back – not an apology, not an offer to send a team of cleaners to blitz the place, not even an acknowledgment of our message the entire weekend! And this was the VIP package that we had paid big money for. The head of the English department confirmed in a company video, that the VIP package was only different in the service that you receive and not the medical quality. There is a 10,000 Euro difference between the standard and VIP package. So, for 10, 000 Euros extra we received a 2-bedroom apartment, with a live-in housekeeper that stayed on the couch with all her stuff including personal items around the lounge (in fact no one even came to collect them and we had to gather them up ourselves and put them out of our sight in the passage cupboard where they are probably still sitting), a repulsively filthy apartment that the housekeeper made even dirtier rather than cleaned. And on the cleaning note, she refused to do our clothes washing as well! In fact all she did was make (out-of-date and dangerously unsafe) meals, watch Ukrainian TV on the couch, talk loudly on the phone and obviously sit on the balcony smoking cigarettes. Kind of defeats the object of having a housekeeper. We later found out that this woman was supposed to double up as the nanny for our babies too! Wow!

We were told on the Monday in no uncertain terms that the staff from the agency do not work on weekends – even for a 50, 000 Euro VIP package! If we had known this, we would have saved our money and bought the budget package instead! *We have found out since, that other IP's are getting the VIP package that we expected but yet we did not receive. I am very happy for those couples receiving good treatment, however, I firmly believe that the agency should have moved us and tried their best to make it up to us as well as the next couples – or at the least we should have been reimbursed the extra money that we spent on the so-called VIP package!*

On the plus side we met our beautiful surrogate in person for the first time. She really was a dream and perfect for us. She was a happy, smiley, positive person who just shone from within, even while 9 months pregnant with our 2 BIG boys! Unfortunately, she couldn't speak English and we couldn't speak any Ukrainian, so all our conversation happened with a translator from the agency. If we were able to speak the same language, I'm pretty sure that we would have been great friends – almost sisters. My friends who have seen pictures of us together say that we look so similar too – even down to the body shape. At that stage she was all twins on her tiny frame. Her warm and loving nature would light up a dark sky and what better oven for our boys to begin absorbing the goodness in life?! In addition to her glowing character, she also glowed on the outside. She ate healthy, exercised and took great care of herself and we could see this without a doubt! She told us that Max responded in leaps when she played music and danced, and we could see that within days of Max being born – he is still such a lover of music and dance. Ultimately, she is the hero of this story and we are forever grateful for our gorgeous angel!

In the 12 days that we waited for our boys to arrive, we explored Kiev by bus, we walked for miles every day from our apartment into town (about a 90-minute walk) and around town, we got a feel for the metro, we did some local sightseeing, sampled a number of restaurants, got surrounded by the pigeon man (details in my blog post – link below), familiarised ourselves with the baby stores in the area and stocked up on more stuff, we met with a few other couples from Australia and the UK who had also turned to Ukraine for surrogacy, we enjoyed some adult beverages and entertainment at the world-famous Buddha Bar, tried to recover from our jetlag (Florida is 7 hours behind Kiev), we had chest x-rays (a requirement to enter the maternity hospital as TB is common in Ukraine) and most of all tried to calm our nerves as I clutched my phone so tightly waiting for "The Call" to say our surrogate was in labour!

CHAPTER 6 – THE BIRTH OF OUR BOYS

From Monday 17 July 2017 (incidentally, this is my hubby's birthday) to 9 am on Thursday 20 July 2017, we dared not to breathe too loudly in case we missed "The Call". I hardly ate. I couldn't sleep. I couldn't focus on much at all. Every few hours I messaged our agency coordinator and our surrogate to find out what was happening – was she in labour, was she in pain, were the boys about to make an appearance?!

At 9 am Thursday 20 July 2017, we decided that we best get our strength up and risk going to the grocery store, which was a half hour walk away. (actually, we found out a few weeks later that we had a little convenience store right in our apartment building!!! And no one thought to tell us this!!). Of course, as Sod's Law goes, about 15 minutes after Vinny left for the shop, "The Call" came! Vinny ran back to the apartment at break neck speed and hurt his ankle, but the trooper kept running through the pain!

We sped to the hospital and were greeted with a bit of a shock at the state of things! The hospital was very tatty and reeked of cigarette smoke. The staff were very rude to us. I was taken to our surrogate who lay on a bed in a white walled room and nothing else – nothing to keep her mind off the pain – not even a picture on the wall! It was like an institution! Down the hall there were eerie screams from other women in labour. It was a surreal experience – like being in an old Alfred Hitchcock film!

One thing I will say, is that the staff seemed to be taking good care of our lady. Well, I say assume, because the language barrier made it impossible to know what they were saying to her but their faces and actions toward her seemed to be of genuine care. This was most important.

Finally, after about 3 hours of her and I trying to communicate with via translating app, calling the agency translator who waited on the surrogate ward with Vinny, hand and face animations and even selfies (for our eyes only though), we were whisked to the delivery room. Part of our VIP package was for us to be present at the birth (although the hospital would only allow me and not Vinny to be present, which the little chicken-S*&t was relieved about ha).

This was an incredible experience and I'm sure there is nothing else like it. This meant so much to me after not being able to carry our babies! Our surrogate was an absolute hero all the way through.

Maximus Vincent Smith was born at 14.05 and Alexei Felix Smith came along 15 minutes later. Both were fully developed, extremely healthy and needed no time in the NICU. While the staff (and that was about 12 people due to there being twins) attended to our surrogate, I floated to the surrogate ward where Vinny waited and 2 hours later we were called to go and see our new baby boys! Nothing felt real that day or at least for 3 months after, especially after so many years of trying, failed treatments and heartaches. We could not believe we were finally parents. Even now 6 months later, I still can't believe how blessed we are with these two treasures! Here's a You Tube video clip of **Our Twins are 2 hours old https://youtu.be/ri4UUKt7rvg**

One thing I was disappointed about was that we were not permitted to do skin-to-skin straight after they were born. The hospital told us not to touch them and we were sent home and told that we could visit them again the next day. This was kind of confusing, as the agency clearly tells people that on the VIP package they could engage in this experience. At this stage we were also not told how they were doing, what tests or meds they were given and when they would be discharged. Our contract also clearly stated that if the babies had to stay in the hospital, we would be put up in a room with them. This seemed to have been a total surprise to them. We found out days later that we were in fact the first VIP couples to request this service and not just that, but that we were only the third VIP couple EVER for the agency.

So, we were the guinea pigs. It's all very well as everyone needs to start somewhere but this should have been conveyed to us instead of making us believe that they were experienced at the service that we were paying them to provide. We also found out that the hospital we used was not one that was usually used and therefore a room wasn't set up for us and the hospital staff were not pro surrogacy which was the reason that they treated us badly. The entire time, right up to the moment we arrived for our babies' birth, we believed that we were getting a private maternity hospital. On the agencies website, they have pictures of a beautiful new maternity hospital they use, and this is the one we thought our boys were going to be born at. Again, we only found out days after their birth, that the hospital on their website does not even exist yet but was still going to be built. We were shocked. It costs roughly $1,000 to have a baby at a private hospital in Kiev and we would have gladly paid this many times over if we had only known! But unfortunately, the agency kept us completely in the dark and never gave us a choice.

On our way to the hospital the following day, a room was quickly made up for us on the surrogate ward. It was tiny and sweltering with a filthy bathroom attached. It was not appropriate for one newborn baby let alone twins! We were overjoyed to be with our little boys but really struggled in that environment. Here's a video I made when we first arrived in the room **– Our Twins are 28 hours old - https://youtu.be/7rikcUbHZig**

The surrogate ward was far from exciting – general hospital corridors, a kitchen and rooms made for 2 people-sharing. The heavily pregnant surrogates seemed to be quite bored which is probably why a few of them smoked cigarettes – nothing else to do all day as they waited to give birth. On the agencies website, it shows a video of where the surrogates stay in the final weeks leading up to the birth – a beautiful hotel with swimming pool in which they do special exercises, go for long leisurely walks in the park, have special cooks that make food according to their cravings and what their bodies need and so on. On this ward, a hospital worker brought big pots of what looked like stew and set them in the kitchen for everyone to have. There was no exercising, no swimming pool and none of the glamour that they show in their website video.

The next few days were amazing and challenging at the same time. We were new parents – new twin parents! We had to learn (doubly) how to change diapers, sterilize and make bottles, calm hours of crying without a clue on how to do that, make sure that they kept breathing and feeding – all this within a hot, dirty and hostile environment in a foreign country where no one spoke our language and didn't care to have us there. The doctors came in and out and did various checks and tests, but no one told us what the tests or what the results were. At night they locked the kitchen and we had to scramble around trying to find someone on duty to explain that we needed water for the newborn bottles!

We were told up to that point was that they do not discharge over the weekend and that's why we could not go home – which was not acceptable. We begged, we pleaded, we demanded to go home with our babies without any more delay. Only after anger and frustrated tears, did they tell us that the babies could not go home with us until our surrogate was discharged as legally she was still considered the mother until the day of discharge when the papers get signed – not before. Of course, we would have understood this if they had been up front and honest with us in the first place! On the plus side, out surrogate stayed in a room next to us, so we saw and spoke to her every day to ensure that she was getting better. She even helped with feeding and rocking the babies when they cried.

Before we left, our surrogate signed all the necessary paperwork needed to obtain the Ukrainian birth certificates. These were arranged by the agency and the hospital. It was a very emotional goodbye and while one driver took our surrogate home, another took us directly to the agency where they took swabs for the DNA test, which is needed for the UK passport application and Parental Order. ** It is important to note here that no matter how many times I explained the importance of baby car seats to our agency, they refused to accommodate us saying that their vehicles were not equipped to carry baby car seats and therefore it wasn't possible for us. Instead, we had to use baby carry cots or bassinets. I was terrified as it certainly did not feel safe especially with the type of aggressive driving that is done by everyone in Kiev – but unfortunately, we had no choice.**

Once back at the apartment we set up camp in the lounge with both babies in one crib for a few weeks until they graduated to their own cribs – and continued to learn about this (twin) parenting thing, how to get by on close to zero sleep, how to go about organizing the mountains of legal paperwork to obtain British passports and how to live with twin babies in this foreign country with its unusual culture and crazy terrain – here's a video of our first outing with the twins where you can see the terrain that I'm talking about **Twins First Outing** https://youtu.be/ho-FLkZOpP8

CHAPTER 7 – FOUR MONTHS IN KIEV WITH INFANTS

As this is not a parenting book, I'm not going to get into our experiences as new (twin) parents, but rather highlight our stay in Kiev with newborns while we waited for the boys' British passports.

At 10 days old we had a gorgeous newborn photo shoot with the very talented and incredible woman, Vita Sovetova of **Sovetoff.Photo (her Facebook page,** where you can see all her beautiful images). She is fantastic with babies and we could not have asked for better pictures or a better photo shoot experience. Just before leaving Kiev, we arranged to do holiday photos with her at the studio and those were just as gorgeous!

Ukraine does not vaccinate their children, which is quite worrying when exposing newborns to people in public and especially to the nannies who come in very close contact with them. ***More of the nanny/ housekeeper saga to follow shortly.

So even though Ukraine does not do vaccinations, the agency offered to arrange these for us. At 2.5 weeks old we were all picked up by the agency driver in the tiniest of cars – me, my 6-foot 5 husband and 2 babies, each in a carrycot (due to no provisions for car seats) and taken to a private medical clinic to get BCG vaccinations. One of the agency translators met us there as there was no English spoken at the medical centre. The paediatrician was very nice and did a full examination on the boys but decided that they could not have their vaccinations that day because 1) they were under weight and 2) she thought that Alexei had a cold because of his snotty nose. A week later the boys' weights were up, and they concluded that Alexei's snotty nose was not a cold but rather something that babies often get from birth, which goes away within a year.

The day after the vaccinations, Alexei didn't seem to be himself at all and towards the evening his body had swollen up like someone with a seafood allergy. I called the agency's 24-hour medical emergency number for help and our manager told as that she would arrange for him to get checked out at a very good private facility where their preemies are often taken care of. A few hours later a car picked me and Alex up with a driver and an agency representative who spoke no English and therefore couldn't even tell me where we were going. We drove for more than an hour in the dark – the driver even got lost and I was frightened. A sick baby, no English, no idea where we were or where we were going. Finally, we got to a building that reminded me of something out of an old film – the ones where the pregnant teenager is sent to be locked up in a remote convent of strict nuns. When the car pulled up, the agency rep phoned someone to come down and unlock the chains from the door. We were ushered in quickly.

Alex was taken from my arms and no one told me anything because no one could speak English. They were very unfriendly and frightening. I didn't know what this place was or where my son was going or when I would see him again. They didn't even want to take his overnight bag of familiar things. I felt panicked. This was no normal hospital that I had ever been to. It was eerie and uncomfortable, and I immediately regretted going there and leaving my baby boy. I cried all the way back to the apartment and didn't sleep that night – my imagination went wild. The next morning the manager sent a car to collect me to go and visit him – but I made my husband go and get Alex. I told him that he was not to leave that institution without my little boy! As I suspected, they didn't want to release him – which is why I sent my giant, military husband in my place. Finally, the hospital gave up, but the manager told us that if we take him, then we are fully responsible for what happens to him from that moment forward. Absolutely. I wanted nothing less!

The following day, Alexei's swelling had gone but both boys seemed out of sorts. They had no energy, struggled to breathe and were off their milk. The last thing I wanted to do was call our agency as I did not want a repeat of that strange institutional encounter. So, I started looking for English speaking doctors. I joined a Kiev expat group on Facebook and asked for doctor recommendations. One of these was **Dr Sam Medical Network (https://doctorsam.ua/en).** I emailed them then spoke to them on the phone and within hours a paediatrician and translator was at our apartment – not that the doctor needed a translator (unlike the agency doctor who claimed she spoke English but kept phoning the translator for every sentence she spoke to us!). The paediatrician confirmed that the boys had a virus – either from the nanny or from the hospital that Alexei had been in! We immediately decided that Dr Sam Medical Network would be our go to paediatricians for the full time that we would be in Kiev – and they never disappointed. I highly recommend them and every one of their staff members. On occasion I also had to see them for my own medical issues – they are a full medical network for all ages with many specialists at their 3 Kiev branches – and they were fantastic with me too!

Throughout the time that we were in Kiev, Dr Sam Medical Network looked after our boys very well. They had check-ups with the paediatrician as well as specialists, even arranged an ultrasound for Max when I suspected that there was something wrong with his stomach because he didn't stop spitting up half his bottle at every feeding. They also specially ordered in vaccinations from Europe. The paediatrician always put my worries to rest when I would annoy him 50 times a week with my questions! He was extremely helpful and accommodating and never brushed me off.

***OK, the nanny story.

As mentioned, the first housekeeper who was also supposed to be the nanny was a flop before the babies even arrived – which is a good thing as she was a complete health & safety hazard!

After finally establishing that we did not want a live-in nanny, the second lady was sent to us to work daily for 8 hours (as per our VIP contract). She seemed nice. She smiled a lot and was gentle with the boys. She took care of them for several days while we ran out to the baby shops and got supplies for them – like a baby swing and more toys. *I recently found out that the agency now provides these things for their VIP customers. We bought these big items and had to pay for extra and over-sized luggage to take them back to the UK &*

America with us.

A big thing that we were not happy with, is the fact that Ukraine still believe in swaddling the babies warmly and then keeping them in heated room of over 30 degrees C. Common Western practice is to keep babies cool – this is especially important for preventing SIDS (sudden infant death syndrome). Western baby care advises a room temperature of between 20 and 23 degrees C and not over 25 degrees. The hospital room where we stayed with the boys was sweltering. The hospital room where Alexei spent the night was sweltering and then this nanny directly disobeyed our instructions to keep the room and babies cool. One day we got back earlier from the shops than expected and this nanny had wrapped them up warm and had purposefully turned off the air-conditioning. Keep in mind, that this was the middle of a very hot summer. Kiev gets up to 36 degrees C in summer and the inside of the apartments are very hot and stuffy. As soon as we walked into the apartment, the nanny quickly scrambled to grab the air-conditioning remote and turn on the cool air. It was stifling and difficult to breathe. This was not a mistake – we had given her definite instructions before we left to make sure that she keep the temp below 25 degrees C. We had even bought a digital room thermometer for her to check and to help her regulate the temp. When we got back on this day, then thermometer read 32 degrees C. This was the main reason that I had to let her go. I couldn't trust her.

But in addition to this, we only found out a week after she was there that she was also the cleaner. Yet the entire week, she had sat on the couch talking or texting on her phone while Vinny had been cleaning the apartment. Not once did she say that she was supposed to clean or offer to clean anything. Most of the time she got to us late and asked to leave early. When we asked the agency to send around someone to clean, they told us that we already had the cleaner – it was the nanny. So, they instructed her to clean, but before she did, suddenly another girl walked into our apartment and sat down at our kitchen table while we were eating!!!! What?! Who does this? Who is this? Why is she here? The nanny/cleaner said this was her friend who was going to help her clean. What?! No asking us or even warning us before-hand why was she sitting at our table? In total shock, Vinny and I went to the park with the boys and returned an hour later to find both gone. Need I say more on this situation? Would *you* be happy with this kind of **VIP** service?

That brings us to nanny/cleaner number three. Within an hour of her being newly in our apartment, she had grabbed Alexei from my arms while I was changing him and proceeded to change his diaper herself but without using a wet wipe or barrier cream – which we use every time. No problem if you don't on your kids, but I expect the nanny to follow my wishes when it comes to my kids. Then she proceeded to tell Vinny to burp Max in the way she wanted him burped and not the way he was doing it. He told her several times that the way he was burping Max was perfectly fine and according to the three main safe methods taught to us by medical professionals. She didn't want to accept this and carried on moaning at him. This was the straw that broke the camel's back and I refused to have her there any longer.

So, after three disastrous nannies/cleaners, we thought it far better to do everything ourselves despite being brand new parents to twins in a foreign country with a foreign language, no family or friends to help and despite having paid for all the services we were not receiving. Doing it ourselves was far less stressful that what we had dealt with already!

I must admit that it was not easy to do it alone. We were very far from town and anyone that spoke English. The closest shop was half hour walk away through underground walkways that was not stroller friendly. The sidewalks were full of potholes which punctured our stroller tyres, as well as great big holes where construction was going on. Taking a taxi or über was also difficult and dangerous as they were not equipped for baby car seats. As a result, we were very much confined to our apartment for the four months.

Vinny's parents came to visit us twice and we had the occasional couple from the UK, Australia and America come and visit us who were also doing surrogacy in Kiev. But other than that, it was a long and isolated existence for all four of us.

In August Vinny had to travel back to America for 2.5 weeks for work. As is was not possible to go to the shops on my own with twins due to no stroller access and because we now had no nanny, I had to have 2 of my girlfriends come over from the UK to help me with a split shift (each came for 10 days). I asked the agency to arrange a driver to collect friend 1 from the airport and our agency manager rudely informed me that the driver for personal use is not part of our package. She quickly kept quiet when I asked her whether I could send her a copy of the contract I signed which clearly states that for the VIP package, the driver is completely at our disposal during our stay in Kiev. In fact, when we were in Kiev for our first visit, that same manager had said that it was only a pleasure for us to request the driver if we wanted to go anywhere to visit or to a restaurant, etc. So, I was fully taken aback when she contradicted herself and our signed contract. Nevertheless, to ensure that we had as little dealings as possible with the agency so as not to get us any more stressed out, we decided to only use über or taxi and not ask the agency for the driver again!

Most of our days were spent trying to stay awake, learning how to be new (twin) parents, answering many emails and messages from people who are following in our footsteps to Kiev for surrogacy, helping our boys with milestones and trying to keep them entertained, going for walks in the park behind our apartments as well as prepping the mountain of paperwork needed for the legalities of our surrogacy situation – prepping and applying for the boys' British passports and UK Parental Order. More on both these points in the following chapters.

So, let's look at our contract again and see what we got out of it…..

ALL INCLUSIVE VIP PACKAGE 49,900 EUROS (ROUGHLY $62,000 OR £44,000)

The Intended Parents

#Accommodation in a separate apartment provided by the clinic - *check*

#All food cooked on premises by a housekeeper to match the standard of food at the hotel accommodation *** *the standard of food cooked did not even match a one-star hotel – complete health hazard and dangerously close to poisonous due to long overdue expiry dates and touching everything in the kitchen with hands that had been in raw meat. Kitchen utensils, including plates, glasses, pots, pans and cutlery had never been washed.*

#Services of a personal driver with a vehicle *** *we were very rudely informed that the driver was not for personal use even though it says in the contract*

#A smartphone and a Ukrainian SIM card for communication *** *After asking several times and already being in Ukraine for nearly a week, we were given a Ukrainian sim card but no phone. We were also not given any credit on the sim card or instructions on how to load the credit – everything was in Ukrainian no English*

#The services of an interpreter throughout the program – *check – these ladies were fantastic!*

#Needed blood tests are performed by a nurse in the apartment where the Intended Parents are staying – *nope we waited at the clinic*

#All medical services needed to achieve pregnancy, including medical examination & tests for Intended Parents throughout the program - *check*

#The Intended Parents are provided with PGD service to detect the possible genetic abnormalities. If needed the sex of a baby may be detected (for medical reasons only) - *check*

#A Surrogate who has had already had a successful previous surrogacy pregnancy and birth *** - *nope this was the first time our lady was a surrogate but as she was so amazing we wouldn't have wanted to swap her anyway!*

#Miscarriage, abortion or death at any time during the program, reattempts will be covered fully by the clinic on this package – *n/a for us thank goodness!*

#In case of premature birth all the expenses related to additional medical treatment and special medical equipment utilization shall be covered by the clinic from the first day of birth – *n/a for us thank goodness again!*

#The Intended Parents can stay in the specially equipped maternity house (hospital) together with a baby *** *nothing especially equipped about this hospital!*

#The Intended Parents are provided with a newborn package – all the things needed to take care of a newborn baby - *check*

#The Intended Parents are provided with a complete physical check-up of the baby by specialists *** - *we had a doctor come around but NO specialists!*

#The Intended Parents are provided with a paediatrician who shall visit the baby every day. A 24/7 phone consultation with a leading English-speaking paediatrician will also be available. If needed the leading paediatrician will visit the baby upon request. *** *The doctor had to keep phoning the translator for every sentence!*

#The services of a babysitter from 9am to 6pm – *yes but you've read about the disasters in this area*

#No additional charge for TWINS - *check*

#Preparation and signing of the Contract between Surrogate and Intended Parents - *check*

#Preparation and signing the Contract between the clinic and Intended Parents - *check*

#Coordination and monitoring of all personal documents throughout the program - *check*

#Coordination and Supervision of the full Surrogacy program until the birth of the baby and the preparation of the necessary documents for the baby to return home with the parents - *check*

#The clinic will provide information via email on the surrogate's pregnancy at least once a month - *check*

#DNA tests to confirm parenthood in a clinic appointed laboratory - *check*

#Submission of the documents concerning the birth certificate of the child to the Ukrainian Civil Registry Office, where the names of the Intended Parents are indicated. Translation and legalization of the birth certificate are also included - *check*

#Assistance to the Intended Parents in obtaining a passport/travel pass in the name of the child - *check*

The Surrogate

>All medical procedures for the Surrogate - *check*

>Psychological and physical testing for the Surrogate to ensure that she is in a fit state for pregnancy and delivery of a healthy baby - *check*

>All ultrasounds and medical care for the Surrogate throughout the pregnancy - *check*

>Weekly check-up by the clinic (by phone or visit) of the Surrogate's health and needs during her pregnancy including any medical examinations – *we assume so but no way to know*

>Medical insurance for the Surrogate in case of unforeseen circumstances – *we assume so*

>Birth of the baby - *check*

>In case of miscarriage, abortion or death *before* 12 weeks, then the clinic will cover the expenses of reattempts - time periods before additional attempts will be determined by the doctor only. – *n/a thank goodness!*

>Transportation, accommodation in a private room and meals for the Surrogate *** - *she was not in a private room but shared.*

>Payment to the Surrogate for pregnancy and birth - *check*

Note the following EXCLUSIONS:

Transportation from own country to Kiev

All the expenses related to the processing of papers by the relevant Embassies and issuance of the travel documents/passports by these authorities

Payment Schedule for the VIP Package

First instalment: **10,000** EUROS - FIRST VISIT TO CLINIC AFTER SIGNING CONTRACTS

Second instalment: **9,900** EUROS - SECOND VISIT BEFORE FERTILIZATION

Third instalment: **10,000** EUROS – AFTER THE 12 WEEK ULTRASOUND

Fourth instalment: **10,000** EUROS - AFTER BIRTH OF THE CHILD BEFORE PAPER PROCESSING

Fifth Instalment: **10,000** EUROS - AFTER RECEIVING BABY'S BIRTH CERTIFICATE & ON DAY OF EMBASSY APPOINTMENT. ANY ADDITIONAL DOCUMENTS REQUIRED BY THE EMBASSY ARE PREPARED AFTER THE FINAL PAYMENT IS MADE. *** *Even though this is what our contract states, we were rudely informed by the agency that they would NOT give us the birth certificates until we had made the final payment!*

A few extra notes about staying in Kiev

*It is not advisable to drink water from the tap. There are some visiting couples who say they had no problems with the tap water but when even the locals don't drink their own tap water, then I am certainly not going to.

In fact, I did one day by mistake and I paid for it by running to the bathroom several times! As part of our package, we had big family sized bottles of water delivered to our apartment weekly for a fee of 21 Hryvnas per bottle. Water is readily available to purchase in all stores.

*Local sim cards with loads of data are very cheap – roughly about $4 for 4G and you can buy these in phone shops (some of the phone shops in the city centre have English speaking shop assistants), on the street and at vending machines throughout the city.

*A good thing to note if you are going to Kiev in winter is that the heating is controlled by the government and is only switched on around 15 October. If you have newborns, you would need to invest in a portable oil heater or similar to keep warm. After a week or two of freezing our butts off we discovered that the apartment had underfloor heating! This was a dream and kept us nice and toasty.

*Speaking of government control – certain websites are not accessible in Ukraine. I'm not sure how they decide to block them and for what reason. I wanted to go onto an American nanny website as well as another surrogacy website in Kiev, but both were blocked.

*The alphabet is Cyrillic which is impossible for us to read unless we have actually learnt it – which I did through 2 free apps – **Memrise** and the best one **Duolingo**. I practiced for about 3 months before we went over – reading, writing and speaking and it made a huge difference especially when it comes to buying something as simple as milk. I always have a chuckle as most people end up buying a few wrong products before they buy milk. Their milk bottles/cartons are not the same as ours and if you do not know the word for milk or how it is written in Ukrainian then you will end up with yoghurt, or buttermilk, or soup or even lemonade as my father in law did! You do get an app in which you can take photos of paragraphs to translate but it's never exact – especially in Ukrainian. In fact, when you want to translate anything it is best to use Russian and not Ukrainian. Although there is some difference in alphabetical letters between the two, they are very similar, and most people can understand both. Usually a hybrid of Ukrainian and Russian is spoken in Kiev.

*Be careful of scammers, tricksters and pick-pockets. You will especially be an easier target if you are with a baby – or two, like my friend and I were. We were each carrying one of my boys in front carriers when we entered an underground pedestrian walkway to cross the road (there are more of these traffic lights or above ground pedestrian crossings), when she suddenly felt a hand in her jacket pocket. She whipped around and caught a young girl in the act of trying to steal her phone from her pocket. We were surrounded by a group of teenagers – something out of Oliver Twist and the street gangs that pickpocketed. They had obviously seen us carrying babies and chatting in English so thought we wouldn't even notice them. Unfortunately for them, they came off second best as my friend let them have it! They quickly ran away from us thank goodness!! Be aware always!

CHAPTER 8 – THE BRITISH PASSPORT APPLICATION FOR YOUR INTERNATIONAL SURROGATE BABIES

You can apply for your baby's British passport as soon as you receive the translated and apostilled Ukrainian birth certificate. Our process went like this:

*When our surrogate was discharged from the hospital, she signed forms relinquishing her rights as the mother. **Only then could our babies be discharged into our care.**

*Once this happened, the agency arranged to register the birth of the babies with us as the parents – this was 2 weeks after they were born. They made an appointment for us to go with a translator to the registration office, where we had to sign various forms and were issued with the birth certificates in Ukrainian. *We are unsure why this took so long, as we know for a fact that other agencies can do this the very day that they are discharged. We suspect it was because it was summer holidays and most staff members were away.*

*Our agency took these forms to be translated and apostilled – this process took another 2 weeks and our agency refused to release them to us until we had made the final payment – even though it states in the contract that the final payment was only due AFTER receiving the birth certificates.

*I then emailed the Passport Application Centre (**hmpo.ukraine@tlscontact.com**) with 3 choices in dates and times for our application interview. Unfortunately, by this time Vinny was away in America so we were delayed by another 3 weeks. The Passport Application Centre sent me a confirmation email the next day.

*Vinny then spent the next few weeks chasing the agency for the required paperwork. They were very slow and kept giving us documents with mistakes and incorrect information – so we had to keep checking and getting them to send us amended documents. It was kind of like they didn't know what they were doing, and we were instructing them on what they should be doing based on our own research.

*As the passport application needed to include both the originals and coloured copies, and because we had twins, Vinny created two files for each baby – one file for originals and one file for the coloured copies, each with an index and coloured tabs for quick and easy reference. Your original documents will be given straight back to you after the clerk has checked them.

*On the day of the interview, the agency driver collected the four of us from our apartment and then went to their office to collect our surrogate, who came with her original identity documents to show the clerks. At the interview, our surrogate and I sat with the babies while Vinny went through all the documentation with the clerk. We did not know at the time, that they also required coloured copies of every page of our passports and not just the photo page. They offered to do this for us for a fee of 10 Hryvnias per page.

*The total time spent at the passport application centre was 90 minutes.

*After the application interview, the clerk gave us a checklist on which they ticked all the documents we gave them. This piece of paper together with original photo ID needed to be taken with for the collection of the passports.

*It is important to note that the passport application centre in Kiev is NOT a British Government property and neither does it have British Government workers. This is a Ukrainian facility that offer to take in the British passport applications on behalf of British citizens. This passport office is also where the passport will be collected again (*not the actual British consulate or embassy*). **The address of this facility is:**

Artem Business Centre
Hlybochyts'ka Street 4,

Kyiv City,

Ukraine, 04050.

Web: https://uk.tlscontact.com/ua

Here is a list of the documents that the clerk at the application centre

asked us for, according to her list:

>Completed application form for each baby

>Completed payment authorization. The fee at the time of our application was £76 per child, which included a courier fee for them to send the printed passports from the UK to Kiev. We needed to fill in a credit/debit card authorization form for this payment.

>Both our original passports PLUS coloured copies of each page of our passports

>Proof of British nationality for both of us – this meant birth certificate for Vinny and naturalization certificate for me.

>Proof of residency in the UK (3 different documents) – this requirement does not appear on the government website, and it was just by chance that we had 3 random documents with us showing our registered UK address.

>2 Passport photos of each baby – one signed at the back by the same person that countersigned the form. *****This one is tricky!** You will need a British professional person who has known you for at least 5 years to countersign the back of the photos and verify that the babies are who you say they are. As the babies are born in Ukraine and you are in Ukraine, your counter signatory would be back in the UK. So, what we did was take our own baby photos, email them to Vinny's parents in the UK who printed them and had them signed, then brought them with when they came to visit. Due to the delay in our application being lodged, the passport photos expired – they must not be older than 1 month! So, we had to redo the photos and this time get them sent to us via courier – Vinny was in the USA at the time, so he had his parents courier the photos to him there and he brought them back with him to Ukraine. Something to watch out for!***

>Surrogacy Agreement

>Babies' birth certificates

>All medical records – antenatal as well as after care

>Copies of surrogate's identity documents

The following documents was part of the list on the British government website, so we insisted that the clerk take these in too, although she was reluctant as they weren't on her list:

+DNA tests

+Document where surrogate relinquishes her parental rights and agree to commissioning parents applying for the babies' passports

+Notarised document confirming that the surrogate was never married

+Letter from the head doctor of the clinic confirming that we were surrogacy clients

+Photographs of us with the babies from their birth to date

*** We figured the more documents we could give them in support of our application, the smoother and quicker the process would go ***

For more information in this regard, visit the following page on my blog www.wheresmystork.com/passport-requirements-for-british-nationals

A week after our application interview, we called the passport office in the

UK to check whether they had taken payment, received our documents and how long we could expect processing to be. They confirmed all had been received, gave us a reference number and instructed us not to call them again until 3 weeks had passed.

Ten days later, we received an email from the passport office in the UK asking us to provide them with the following information:

*Surrogate's full home address

*Our current Ukrainian address

*A letter on a hotel or clinic letterhead, translated into English, confirm that we are staying at the address we are claiming to be staying at

*Dates when we might not be in the Ukraine and therefore not available for the final interview

All the above needed to be filled in on their official forms which were emailed to us and which we needed to email back to them. Their message also stated that we would hear from them again in around 10 weeks with information about the final interview and that we should not contact them again before the 10 weeks have passed.

Four weeks after our application interview, we received a date for the final interview which was to be a month later.

Nine weeks after our initial application interview, Vinny attended the final passport interview (the boys and I did not need to be there). This was a half hour video conference call with the UK in which they confirmed Vinny's identity, history and random facts.

We called the passport office in the UK several times to find out how the processing was going and when we could expect the passports. A week after the final interview they told us that the passports were being printed and we could expect them in about 7 to 10 working days.

A week after this telephone call, we received an email from the passport application centre in Kiev advising that our passports were ready for collection. The following morning Vinny ran all the way to the centre to collect them!

Quick Look Summary of the Passport Process for British Citizens (based on our experience)

1 Make sure your marriage certificate is apostilled before you go!

2 If wife's name on her passport is the same as her married name, then she she will need to get an affidavit signed by a notary confirming that the person born Mary Jones is the same person who is now Mary Smith after marriage.

3 Once your baby is discharged from the hospital, your agency will arrange to obtain the Ukrainian birth certificate. This should happen the day of discharge.

4 You will need to go with the agent to the Registration Office in Kiev and sign the paperwork and the birth certificate will be issued immediately. With some agencies this has happened on the day of discharge from the hospital while other agencies have taken a few weeks.

5 Your agent will then arrange for this birth certificate to be translated and apostilled. Again, this will take from a few days to a few weeks depending

on the efficiency of your agency.

6 Once you have these documents, you can email the Visa Application Centre with your preferred dates for your application interview.

7 Attend the interview where you will hand over all your original documents to check and they will take in all your coloured copies.

8 Call the passport office in the UK to confirm receipt of documents, payment and obtain a reference number.

9 Await for correspondence from the UK Passport office either asking for further information or confirming your final interview date.

10 Attend Final interview. Roughly 8-16 weeks after application.

11 Await for passports. Ours arrived a week after the final interview.

A point to keep in mind too, is that your baby born via surrogacy in Ukraine will not automatically get a Ukrainian passport, so you will have to apply for the passport of the country of which the biological parent is a citizen.

We spent the time between our passport application and receiving our passports, to focus on getting our UK Parental Order started.

CHAPTER 9- THE UK PARENTAL ORDER PROCESS FOR YOUR INTERNATIONAL SURROGATE BABIES

The UK passport will mean your baby is a UK citizen and will enable your baby to travel internationally.

However, there is one more step for UK parents of babies born via surrogacy to follow to have full parental rights – the Parental Order. UK Surrogacy Law states that the woman who carries and gives birth to a baby regardless of whether she is genetically related to the baby or not, is the mother. If the woman is married or has a live-in partner, that partner is also considered the father of the baby and not the genetic father. This is UK Surrogacy Law and is a requirement whether your surrogate baby was born in the UK or in another country. To be recognized by the UK as the full and legal parents of your surrogate baby, the intended parents need to apply for a Parental Order (PO). Without this Parental Order, you will not be able to renew your children's passports without the surrogate's signature or make major life decisions regarding their health or education. You will also be faced with legal complications in the unfortunate event of divorce or death.

In Ukraine, yes, the names of both intended parents are immediately put onto the birth certificate. However, the UK does not recognise this. Once the Parental Order has been issued, they will issue a new British birth certificate.

Quick Look Summary of the Process

*Prepare initial application pack – not less than 6 weeks after your baby is born.

*Send this application pack together with your court fee to the Central Family Court in London.

*The court will stamp your application, assign a case number and send you copy together with a form that must be given to the surrogate to sign, which you will need to return to the court.

*The court will assign a Parental Order worker called a CAFCASS representative to your case who will get in touch with you to find out more about your family dynamic, how and why you ended up doing surrogacy and visit you at your home in the UK to observe your interaction with your children and check their general welfare.

*The court will send you a date and time for your first court appearance (directions hearing).

*The court will also give you a date by which they expect to see your statement and all the evidence in support of your application.

*After their visit, the CAFCASS reporter will prepare a report to present to the court and make a recommendation about whether a parental order should be made or not.

*For international surrogacy, the application will be heard by a specialist High Court Judge, which follows very formal proceedings and will scrutinize your evidence and statement.

NOTE

The above summary is not necessarily the exact order of things. Each situation is slightly unique, and your case will be dealt with according to your specific situation. As an example, you might be appointed a CAFCASS worker before your hearing date or you might be appointed one only at your first hearing.

Now let's look at the process and documentation in more detail:

Before you do anything else, you need to make sure that your surrogacy situation complies with the <u>UK legal surrogacy requirements for a parental order</u>:

#Legally married heterosexual couple – this is a Ukraine surrogacy law requirement anyway

#Conception must have taken place artificially via fertility treatments – this is a given

#The child must be genetically related to at least one of the intended parents – this is also a Ukrainian surrogacy requirement. DNA evidence must be submitted to the court.

#The application must be lodged no later than 6 months after the child's birth

#The child must be living with the intended parents at the time of application (for example, you cannot apply if your baby is older than 6 weeks but still in the NICU)

#No money can be exchanged other than reasonable expenses – it is recommended to get affidavits, translated, signed by the surrogate and notarized, confirming the monthly amount received for expenses as well as a lump sum for inconveniences while pregnant with the twin boys. You should also keep track of the money paid over to the agency and surrogate and be ready to present these to the Judge. A breakdown of expenses should be obtained from the clinic in writing to present to the court, as well as information on your surrogate's standard of living, previous earnings and occupation.

#There must be a surrogacy agreement signed by the intended parents and the surrogate

#Full consent by the surrogate to the making of the parental order – freely given in an appropriately translated and notarised document not less than 6 weeks from the birth of your baby otherwise it will be null and void.

#At least one of the intended parents must be domiciled in the UK. Domiciled means to call the UK your permanent home even if you temporary live in another country. You must be able to satisfy the court through evidence and statements that you have full intentions of returning to the UK to live there permanently and then it will be up to the judge to decide whether you will be considered domiciled in the UK.

The Initial Parental Order Application Pack

@Complete **C51 Court Form** and a copy of this form with a translation must be provided to the court to officially serve to your surrogate.

@Completed **A101A form** (Agreement to the making of a parental order in respect of a child) – **Section 54** must be translated into your surrogate's home language and she must sign it in the presence of a notary.
@A copy of each child's birth certificate translated into English.

@A copy of your marriage certificate.

@A cheque for the Court Fee. It was £235 at the time of our application but this can change, so phone them to confirm costs. Also, as we do not use cheques, they allowed us to make payment over the phone with our bank card.

Send the above application pack to:
The Central Family Court London

First Avenue House

42-49 High Holborn

London

WC1V 6NP

Court phone number: +44 (0) 207 421 8954

Application Process

*The court will stamp your application, give it a case number and send you a copy of it together with a **C52 Section 54 Acknowledgement Form**.

*This C52 Form which must be translated into the surrogate's home language and signed by her in front of a notary and returned to the court as soon as possible.

* The court will send you notice of your (directions) hearing date, as well as appoint a court representative to contact you, visit you in your home with your children and write a report on their visit to present to the court.

*The court could ask you to send your statement / argument and all your evidence before your hearing so that it can be assessed. For international surrogacy, a High Court Judge will preside over the case.

*During the directions hearing, the court could ask for additional evidence or argument and set a date for the final hearing at which your Parental Order is finalised.

The entire process could take anywhere between 4 and 12 months.

Your Statement/ Argument to present to the court

@Set out who you both are individually, as a couple and your backgrounds.

@Explain your path to surrogacy – what led you to it and why you chose Ukraine.

@Explain how you satisfy all the legal requirements for a Parental Order.

@Talk about your current relationship with your children.

@Describe if and how you plan to tell your children about how they entered the world. *(The UK courts are fully in support of being completely transparent with your children).*

@Talk about the future plans for your children – living arrangements, current and future education, what provisions you have made in the case of separation, divorce, severe injury to or death of either of you.

@List the evidence that you are submitting in support of your application.

Your evidence to present to the court

#DNA reports (the court may ask you to provide DNA reports from a governmental approved testing facility)

#Signed joint Surrogacy Agreement between us as Intended Parents, the Surrogate and the Agency/Clinic.

#Signed, translated, notarized and apostilled document confirming the compensation paid to surrogate. *(This is one of the most important pieces of evidence that the court asks for)*

#Signed, translated, notarized and apostilled document confirming surrogate's agreement to the making of a parental order (Section 54 of the Human Fertilisation Act).

#Ukrainian birth certificates for each child, translated and apostilled.

#Medical, birth and hospital certificates for each child, translated and apostilled.

#Marriage certificate.

#Both of your birth certificates.

#Surrogate's passport.

#Surrogate's confirmation that she has never been married, translated, notarized and apostilled. *(Also an important piece of evidence)*

#Certificate of Naturalisation if applicable.

#Bank statements showing payments to the agency/clinic and surrogate during the surrogacy.

#Any additional documents you feel will help your case, such as your personal fertility medical records.

More information can be found on the official UK government website:

www.cafcass.gov.uk/grown-ups/parents-and-carers/surrogacy/

Note:

On 12 March 2018, we had a visit from lovely our Cafcass case worker at Vinny's parents' home in the North East of England, where we staying while in the UK. Her job was to check that the boys were well taken care, developing well, interacting well with us as parents and also how they were being received and treated by the rest of the family. She asked why we decided to do surrogacy in Ukraine, what our experience was like, what life was like where we lived in Florida, the boys' interests and how we plan to tell them about their origins. The UK courts like to see that intended parents will tell their children how they came about so that there are no shocks later which could be detrimental to their wellbeing.

Of course, I have always been a very open person since the start of our fertility journey. I have. I have documented practically every detail in my blog and book, on my Facebook pages and on the boys' Facebook profile. Therefore, there will never be any secrecy to their origins and they will know from the earliest age, how much they were wanted and loved before thy even arrived and of course, even more so as they grow in size and in our hearts. This is a HUGE plus to the court granting a Parental Order.

Our amazing Cafcass case worker, drew up and submitted her report to the court the next day with a humble request for us to conclude everything in one court appearance instead of the usual two court appearances, due to us living in the USA.

On 15 March 2018, we went before the wonderful High Court Judge in Middlesbrough, who confirmed that we had prepared a fantastic and detailed statement, that all our evidence was exceptionally organised with nothing missing and that my blog (which he had explored the night before) was impressive.

We were ecstatic to hear him say that due to the outstanding job of our Cafcass case worker, as well as the point I mention above, he doesn't need to delay in granting us our Parental Order!

We will forever be grateful to that sweet and kind judge and to our most amazing case worker – words are just not enough to express our gratitude.

CHAPTER 10 – TIPS FROM THOSE WHO HAVE ALREADY BEEN THROUGH THE PROCESS

@Join a surrogacy group beforehand, saves considerable time and nothing like hearing others' experiences. The best Facebook group for support and information is **IP Surrogacy Support Ukraine**. You will be asked to answer questions and prove that your profile is legit.

@Ask many questions if you are unclear about anything.

@Do your due diligence – research every possible angle and find answers to every question you can think of no matter how big or small.

@Be very very very patient!

@It's a stressful process but if you take it day by day it will be much easier.

@Many Ukrainian agencies offer current, past or future clients substantial kickbacks to promote their agency. If it seems too good to be true – it probably isn't true but merely a "sales" ploy.

@Be critical! Good enough is not good enough in surrogacy where you must rely on other people. Service must be excellent. Not only for yourself but especially for the surrogate's health which means a healthy baby for you at the end of your journey.

@Realize it's not going to go as smoothly as doing it in the US but the price is way less!!

@I would say have realistic expectations. I think I expected it to work the first time being that I had a young donor and surrogate, but that wasn't the case. Surrogacy is luck, hope and Faith. You roll the dice playing to win.

@Cheap cost doesn't have to mean cheap service. Things are not going to be the same as in the US but that doesn't mean sacrifice. Make sure things are as good as they can be for the safety of your baby. There are agencies that can make the experience wonderful and those who you will get what you pay for. Do your research so you will know what to expect.

@Check out potential areas where you may stay for the next and longer visit e.g.: when you may be picking up your precious new family member (ask your agency to show you areas that they recommend if they haven't already offered) include apartments, parks, shopping centres, metro etc if you have time. It's is very different travelling for a short vs longer stay.

@Make sure you are well-read and that you are ahead of the stage and have a Plan B. And be patient. It's all about time and money until you will get pregnant and/or can go home with your baby!!!

@Other than being patient and positive (but also understand that is still IVF, so maybe prepare yourself for both possible outcomes)..., maybe trust your guts... When something doesn't feel right, it probably isn't, so don't hesitate to speak up for yourself. It's not the time and place to be afraid of seeming to be nagging or needy.

@Ensure you and your partner are in it together as much as each other and it's a joint decision all the way. The journey is not easy but is possible with no guarantee. Don't hurt your relationship along the way as there will be days where you do feel like the world is against you! Don't forget to treasure what you already have too.

@Document/keep a trail of everything. You never know what the Embassy will ask for.

@Be patient - there are going to be a lot of highs and a lot of lows throughout the journey!

@Work with an agency and clinic you trust as there are times when you just have to let go and trust the people you are working with. One thing that has taken me by surprise is the amazing people I have met along the way - without the support of others who are also doing Surrogacy it would have been a very lonely and isolated journey.

@I would add that we must get a lawyer's advice on possible legalities and paperwork to bring baby home BEFORE signing contracts with the agency. Visit the clinic and check them out, observe how the agency and clinic treat the surrogates and how happy your surrogate is with them. If you're taking an all-inclusive package-ask even more questions before signing the contract.

@Women must know that once your surrogate is pregnant you will feel like an expectant dad who doesn't even get to see the baby bump. LOL!

@Learn to let go and trust the experts.

@Along the way you will meet angels, including perfect strangers, who spend their time helping you and offering love even when the benefit to them is zero and they don't expect anything in return. Their generosity is amazing... and on the flipside you will meet ignorant people even within your friends and family who are not supportive or make hurtful comments. I am working on a philosophy of not sweating the stupidity of others and not having my happiness marred by them. Still working on it.

@Be prepared to stress. If you thought IVF was stressful that is nothing compared to the stress of surrogacy. Nothing is in your control. It can be very consuming mentally and emotionally before you even get a BFP.

@When travelling back home with your one or two babies, consider taking the **VIP service at Boryspil Airport https://kbp.aero/en/infra/vip**–sperate entrance, baggage, security, check-in and personal service all the way, including help with your carry-on bags right to the gate or plane. It takes all the stress out of travelling with an infant and worth the price!

@Take a portable coloured printer with you to Kiev to print out all the documents you will need for the passport application. British IP's will need a coloured copy of all their documents including every page of their passport. A portable, coloured printer is inexpensive and will save you so much trouble and time!

@Infant passport applications will need photos. It's not an easy task. What helped us was **www.idphoto.com**. Put a white sheet behind your baby. Snap away. Upload to site. Auto crop and resize, then download and print onto photo paper!

@Consider brushing up on your Russian before leaving home through some useful and free language apps, like **Duolingo** and **Memrise**. In these apps you can learn to read, speak and write so by the time you get to Kiev you won't feel completely lost. Remember that very little English is spoken there.

CHAPTER 11 - FAQ'S

Can I do surrogacy in Ukraine if I'm considered "too mature" for my own pregnancy? There is no upper age limit in Ukraine but for surrogacy there must be a legitimate medical reason not just age.

Can you use a sperm donor?

That would depend on the agency/clinic.

Can you use a donated embryo? No, one parent must be biologically related to the child.

Can we ship our embryos from our home country? Most agencies/clinics do allow this, but some don't. Do your research.

Are egg donors anonymous? Yes, but you will be able to see pictures.

Do you need a visa for Kiev? – depends on the country of your passport. British, Europeans and Americans don't need one for up to 90 days, but Australians do.

The best way to get around Kiev? – walking, metro or über. As of October 2017, the Metro will cost 5 UAH per ride regardless of where you are travelling within Kiev. This is roughly $0.19! Visit **Kiev4tourists - www.kiev4tourists.com** for detailed info. The über can be frustrating as many drivers are new and don't know their way around town. Often a long waiting time and many lost trips. Most über drivers cannot speak English. Taxi's cost roughly 3 x more and often like to take advantage of tourists. Neither übers or taxis are equipped for baby seats but are better than the metro which is extremely crowded most days but especially in the winter months.

What cost of living can we expect as international IP's? Ukraine is one of the cheapest countries in Europe to visit. Accommodation, transport, food and clothes are many times cheaper than other countries. As an example, you can get a very good meal with drinks in a top restaurant for as little as 12 US Dollars a person or 10-mile ride in an über could cost less than 10 US Dollars. More information on **Expats Ukraine - www.expatua.com**

Can you consume the tap water in Kiev? Some foreigners have and say there's nothing wrong with it, but most don't. Even the locals drink bottled water which is widely available.

How many times do you need to visit Ukraine doing the surrogacy? That depends on the clinic as well as whether you are using own or donor eggs. Usually between one and three visits.

Are the parents permitted in the birthing rooms? Some clinics allow the mother to be present at the birth depending on whether the surrogate herself has given consent or not. However, no fathers are allowed in the birthing room at any time.

What level of contact will there be with the surrogate? Again, that depends on the policy of the agency as well as your preference. Some agencies allow you to choose your won surrogate after interviewing several ladies over skype and then you are welcome to keep as much contact as you like. Other agencies allow minimum contact such as our agency who chooses the surrogate for you and then will only allow you to meet her from 12 weeks pregnant. There have also been IP's who have not any contact with their surrogate at all as per the surrogate's request.

Are the egg donors anonymous? Yes. You will usually be able to see a photo and personal details such as height, weight, education and interests.

What are the hospitals like and is there a choice? There are a range of government and private hospitals and most agencies will give you a choice between two. Unfortunately, we were not given that choice with our agency. The government hospitals are basic and the staff are generally not supportive of surrogacy but there are those IP's who have had great experiences.

Other medical care? **Dr Sam Medical Network** has three branches throughout Kiev. Their service in every department is excellent and they will ensure that your baby has the best care in those first few week or months (depending on the length of your stay).

Can I get my baby vaccinated? Ukraine do not do vaccinations, so you will need to request these especially. Some clinics obtain the vaccines from India or China. **Dr Sam Medical Network** obtain theirs from Europe.

Can we request breastmilk from our surrogate? This is not possible in Ukraine and the surrogates will be given medication to dry up their supply quickly.

Can we arrange cord blood banking in Ukraine? If you are with the right agency, they can arrange to do this for you via a kit that has been shipped in from Europe or America and then ship it to your country.

CHAPTER 12 – THE BABY LIST – WHAT TO TAKE, WHAT YOU CAN GET IN KIEV & OTHER TIPS

Based on Personal Experience

*Nappies (Diapers)

We found out that Pampers nappies are different around the world. We took a stack of diapers with us from America (an entire suitcase worth!) but because we were there for so long, we ran out. The Pampers in Ukraine did not fit as well or smell as nice as those we had taken with. For the fit we found that Huggies was better. You will go through piles of nappies especially with twins. Newborn nappies are specially designed to fold down under the umbilical stump so these are important. We took all our newborn nappy supply with us, but we did run out and struggled to find newborn size (especially Pampers and Huggies) in the supermarket. I would recommend that you take as many newborn and size 1 nappies as you can – these will be used the most. For those staying a little longer, buy size 2 there as they will not be in them for long (a little tip from a friend – thank you Miriam – and my boys proved that to be the case. They hardly used the 2's.)

*Wet Wipes

You will go through these quicker than you can say 'poop'! We bought these in Ukraine and our boys only liked Pampers Sensitive.

*Wipes Warmer

For the first two months our boys hated the cold and they used to cry every time we used the wet wipes (even though we were in the middle of a hot summer at the time!), so I got my hubby to bring a wipes warmer back from the USA. By the time he got back, the boys were over their fussiness about the cold and we didn't end up using it at all.

*Burp Cloths

You will go through many of these in the early months as babies tend to spit up a lot! In my opinion, you can never have too many of these soft muslin cloths. Take with you.

*Pacifiers

You can get these in Kiev at various baby stores, but our boys are fussy and will only use the Tommee Tippee brand which we struggled to find in Kiev, so Vinny had to bring from America. They mostly stock Nuby and Avent. My advice is to get a few different brands and see what your baby prefers before you buy in bulk– believe me, they will let you know exactly what they like and don't like!

*Swaddlers

We took several swaddlers (2 each) and swaddling cloths (2 each) with us which we used a lot during the newborn stage. The swaddlers with stretchy or muslin material are easier to use but we couldn't see any of these in Kiev. They tend to use just big pieces of cotton material.

*Blankets

Due to the risk of SIDS (sudden infant death syndrome), it is highly advisable not to allow your newborn to have any blankets (or anything at all) in the crib or anywhere else when you are not watching to ensure safety. We took two baby blankets each that we would use in the stroller and in their little bouncy chairs.

*Clothing

There is no shortage of shops selling all sorts of baby gear from very cheap to top brands. We ended up taking far too many clothes. Firstly, you won't really know what size your newborn will wear until he or she is born. We had a bunch of newborn clothes that were already too small from day one. We also underestimated how fast babies grow, meaning it is not a good idea to have too many outfits in one size. You can leave behind any outfits that need to go over the head – this is difficult in the first months. Also leave behind two pieces like a top and pants, as the tops ride up and newborns get cold quickly. We found the easiest outfits for all concerned was **full baby grows** – long sleeves with **built in mittens** and long legs with feet, that either **zip up** or have **press studs** (not buttons!). We tried separate mittens, but they kept getting them off and ended up scratching their little faces. Babies are born with sharp claws! Also have a few short sleeved and no legs baby grows for hot days as you don't want the baby to be too hot either. Optimal temperature of the room that baby is kept in especially at night is between 20 and 23 degrees C.

Other than that, you might need a few **hats** depending on the season, a few pairs of **socks** and **bibs**. The bibs that we use are the ones on which you can attach a pacifier. They are called **Zury Oval Bibs** and we bought them off **Amazon**. We still use them now and the boys are 7 months. Now we attach a pacifier and as well as a teether to them. You can never have too many of these either as you constantly want to change them for clean ones.

*Sleeping

Sleep sacks did not seem to be popular anywhere in Kiev, so we were lucky that we had taken some with us. I would say take 2 per baby, long and short sleeve.

We had **cribs, crib mattresses** and **crib sheets** provided within our agency package, but others have either taken travel basinets or baby cocoons. Alternatively, you can rent these from **Baby Service Ukraine - www.babyservice.ua/baby_equipment_rental**, who offer a full range of baby equipment.

Large disposable changing pads are good to put down under the sheet to protect the mattress and under the baby to protect the sheet. We used a lot of these, as accidents and a lot of leaks of spit up happens at that age.

It's always good to have a **humidifier** in a baby's room but especially in Kiev as the air is very dry and could cause nosebleeds and congestion. We bought a cool mist humidifier from the **Stokke** baby shop in the **Cosmopolite Mall - http://cosmopolite-kiev.com/hotel/cosmopolite**. We took it with us to the UK but then could not bring it to America due to the difference in power voltage. We now have a Vicks vapour humidifier which works even better for Alex as he was born with a very congested nose that only started to clear around 5 months old.

White noise. This is extremely helpful for newborns and we still use white noise in the boys' room now. We bought a *shusher* on Amazon in the USA but then we discovered a fabulous app which have everything from the sound of a heartbeat in the womb, to cars, vacuum cleaner and rain. Our boys like a certain sound for a while and then like a change. The app is called Sound Sleeper: Whitenoise. What's great is that it has a 'listen mode', so when your baby stirs it will automatically switch on for a certain amount of time. We used the portable *shusher* in the stroller which was handy.

Baby Monitor. We brought one from the USA.

Nightlight for baby's room. This we bought in Kiev.

*Bath time

Baby baths you can get in Kiev along with various baby **safety nets** to put onto the bath.

Baby bath thermometer is important to ensure the water is not too hot. You can get these there.

Baby soaps and **shampoos** you can get there, although none of it is in English.

Wash cloths we struggled to get so Vinny brought back from America.

Baby towels are limited and the ones we did find were pricy, so I would suggest you take from home.

A **changing pad and/or** changing station is always helpful. We found a wonderful changing station by accident at Mothercare in the centre of Kiev which we brought home and still use now. It came equipped with a bath inside (although they outgrew that quickly), drawers, ledges and various divisions to put everything you need for nappy changing and more. It's also portable which is great as you can move it around the apartment as you need!

Disposable nappy bags. We couldn't find any that were the right size and scented, so Vinny's parents brought from the UK when they came to visit.

Nappy creams are available everywhere but none in English.

Nails. Babies are born with sharp claws and they tend to scratch their own faces due to lack of coordination. Cutting a baby's nails is one of the most difficult tasks so I recommend an electronic baby nail file, like the **Zoli**

Buzz B or similar available on **Amazon**. They work fantastic and my boys like the feeling – like a little massage.

*Medicines

Gripe water is not available in Ukraine. Max was colicky, so we relied on gripe water a lot. We were warned beforehand, so we took a big supply with us. The main ingredient is fennel which is available in pharmacies, but the language barrier makes it difficult to purchase.

Infacol you can get in Ukraine and it's the same as the one found in the UK.

Probiotics and Vitamin D are available in pharmacies, but you may want to take with English instructions.

Nasal spray/ saline solution was another big thing for us with our Alex's snotty and blocked nose from birth. We found that the saline solution in Ukraine did nothing for him. The ones from the **USA** and UK work much better.

Aspirators such as the NoseFrida are available in Ukraine in all pharmacies and baby shops.

Digital Thermometer are also available in all pharmacies and baby shops.

*Feeding

For UK and Australian citizens and anyone else who needs to stay in Kiev for such a long time, it is not a good idea to take **formula** with you. It is impossible to say beforehand what formula will agree with your baby. We had to change Max's formula many times before we found one that his system would tolerate. It would have been a complete waste if we had taken a few months' worth of formula with us. There are many major formula brands and one of those should work until you get home to something more familiar.

Bottles are available in Kiev, but it depends on which ones you want to use. I love Dr Brown's, which have the anti-colic inserts that can be taken out when you don't need them anymore. We couldn't find any Dr Brown's in Kiev. It is advisable to take around 6 per baby. The best **Dr Browns is the wide neck 8 or 9 inch**. As a tip, if you are going to take Dr Brown's bottles then get the travel caps as well to avoid spillage when transporting or warming the bottles.

Bottle sterilizers can be either microwave or electrical. At home I use the Dr Brown's electrical one because its made to fit the Dr Brown's bottles. Over in Kiev, we used the microwave sterilizer but not all apartments will have a microwave. You can buy the Tommee Tippee one in Ukraine, but I didn't see a Dr Brown's.

Bottle warmers are handy. We use the Dr Brown's – again because its made to fit all the Dr Brown's bottles. It is not advisable to warm the bottles up in a microwave because it creates hotspots and can burn a sensitive little mouth. Take from home.

We took the Tommee Tippee bottle prep machine to make the bottles. Put formula in, move dial to the number of ounces you need, press button once for your shot of hot water to kill the germs that could be lurking in the powder, press button again and there we go – a finished bottle, which can be refrigerated for 24 hours. It comes in handy for the first few months, especially with twins. Grab a ready-made bottle from the fridge and warm in the bottle warmer. Formula can be kept at room temperature for 2 hours maximum if not drunk from yet and 1 hour maximum if it has been drunk from.

Bottle drying rack – and you guessed it – we use the Dr Brown's because it fits the bottles well. Take with you.

Baby safe dish washing liquid is available in supermarkets in Kiev.

Bottle brush to clean the bottles well as formula tends to stick.

Boppy pillows we bought there also at the Stokke shop in the Kosmopolit Mall. These are good for feeding especially with twins.

*On the Go

Prams/Strollers can be hired from **Baby Service Ukraine**. The terrain is very rough in Kiev and not stroller friendly at all. If you plan to take your own stroller be prepared for it to possibly break. The locals have strollers specifically designed for their terrain, which is why it is advisable to rent one.

Baby carriers are advisable due to the above-mentioned point. There are many underground walkways with stairs and no proper ramps, so a good baby carrier will be a lifeline. Again, you can hire from Baby Service Ukraine or if you plan to babywear at home you can already invest in a decent one that doesn't hurt your back as much, such as **Ergo** or **Tula**.

A **carry cot** will be used in most cars as baby car seats are popular. My agency could not provide one at all and told us that we could not hire one as they were not prepared to put them in their cars. Also, if you are going to be travelling my über or taxi, the carry cot might be the safest bet. These can be bought from the big Baby Department Store in Kiev for around $25.

Sterilizer tablets such as Milton will be handy when travelling.

Travel change mat for nappy changes on the go – the bigger the better to cover a wide area if you must change in a public place.

I recommend using a **backpack nappy bag**, especially if you have twins as it will be easier to carry around and your weight can be even distributed on both shoulders – really helps when you have some shopping to put into it as well!

*Leisure Time

Full size baby swing. We found a Graco one at a good price at the Baby Department Store. Max loved it and we brought it home with us to America. At 7 months, they don't swing anymore but still use the chair!

As we had two babies, we also picked up a **cheap bouncy chair** at Walmart for roughly $25 which we took over and then brought back and which they also still use.

Crib mobile we bought there. Remember to get black and white as babies don't see colour for the first few weeks.

Baby play mat/ activity gym we bought there. This play mat will be used often for that all-important tummy time.

Baby Einstein DVD's available on **Amazon** will be a life saver when you need to do some work, gather documents or make bottles. They won't be too interested in the first month but as they grow so will their love for it!

English movies for you to watch.

CHAPTER 13 – HELPFUL LINKS

AGENCIES used by previous IP's who were happy with the service & outcome

Fertility Solutions International - www.fertilitysolutionsinternational.com

Lotus Surrogacy - http://lotusukraine.com

New Life Agency - www.newlifeukraine.com

New Hope - http://surrogacyukraine.com/8-main

Successful Parents Agency - http://successful-parents.com

Tammuz - http://www.tammuz.com

Apostille UK documents –

https://www.gov.uk/get-document-legalised

Official UK government to get your documents Apostilled such as your marriage certificate which is a requirement for obtaining your baby's Ukrainian birth certificate.

Baby Equipment Rentals -
http://www.babyservice.ua/baby_equipment_rental

It often makes more sense to rent items that are big, bulky or heavy. Many previous IP's have used this company before for bassinets, cribs and strollers.

Dr Sam Medical Network - https://doctorsam.ua/en

A complete network of medical professionals dealing with children and adult patients, with advanced facilities and technology. English speaking.

Families Through Surrogacy -
http://www.familiesthrusurrogacy.com

This is a non-profit organisation that aims to unite all involved in surrogacy in a positive and enlightened way. Sam Everingham, the founder, works hard to gather intelligence around the globe through personal visits at facilities, conferences, interviews, arranges discounted rates and makes sure that everyone benefits. Everyone who has dealt with Sam only speaks very highly of him.

IP Surrogacy Support Ukraine

The number one Ukraine support group on **Facebook** filled with more information on doing surrogacy in Ukraine than you can imagine! Think of a question, put it in the group's search bar, press enter and there you have instant access to a goldmine of research that's already been done for you — agencies, hospitals, flights, restaurants, tourist attractions, accommodation, tips for travelling with infants, shipping embryos and much more.

Sovetoff.Photo - https://www.facebook.com/sovetoff.photo

Vita Sovetova is an incredibly beautiful person inside and out, amazing with babies and a very talented photographer. I cannot give her enough praise. We are so happy to have the privilege of connecting with her and having our gorgeous newborn and holiday photos taken by her. Her English is great too!

CONCLUSION

In a recent BBC news article, it reported that Surrogacy in Ukraine has grown 1000% since opening its doors in 2015! That is a mind-blowing increase. With this rise, there is already a surge of agencies that will be scammers and steal your money, others that will treat their surrogate ladies like sub-species and those that will try to squeeze as many pennies out of desperate couples eager to fulfil their baby dreams.

The most important thing that you need to do is RESEARCH! Do not go for the cheapest agent. Do not go for the agency that individuals are pushing you to go for. Many agencies, such as the one that we used, offer their current, future and past clients a kickback for promoting them. These kickbacks are substantial amounts of money or huge discounts on their surrogacy packages – sometimes even free surrogacy – to promote the agency regardless of any negative feedback. How do I know this? Because this was offered to me too and at first, I was ecstatic at the thought of the money that I could make but once I compared my personal values to those of the company I was going to represent, I realised that these values were not align at all and I chose to be true to myself and my love for helping other people versus money. Watch out for these individuals and agencies. They are motivated by (your) money and not your welfare, the welfare of your surrogate and not the welfare of your baby. BEWARE!

When we started our surrogacy journey, I could not find another person to connect with who was also going to Ukraine let alone the same agency as myself. If I had access to all the information that is now out there and growing at an incredible rate, we would certainly have spent more time going through all the pros and cons and everything in between. If you are starting now, you are extremely lucky – use everything to your advantage. The information in this book is only a fraction of what you can now find but I hope it is a good start for you. Read, speak to people, join good and VARIED Facebook support groups – not only ones that promote any agency above others.

I will end off by reminding you, that this was a look at my personal experience. Everyone's experience is unique based on a plethora of factors coming together. While I have regrets about aligning myself with the agency, I have absolutely no regrets about pursuing surrogacy in Ukraine and my gorgeous and perfect little boys are all our mommy and daddy dreams come true. I have no disappointment in our surrogate as a person – I would not have wanted anyone else – as a carrier of our precious cargo and as someone who will forever be a part of our lives in some positive way or other. She is truly the star of this show!

Would we do it again? Just to be clear, we are completely fulfilled with our two boys and not planning another surrogacy journey. But if we wanted to, then yes, Ukraine is still a good choice, but we would obviously choose another agency – one of these mentioned above due to the exceptional service that our friends have received there.

I wish you all a wonderful and successful surrogacy journey.

Love, Bianca